# BASICS OF HEALTH CARE PERFORMANCE IMPROVEMENT

## *A Lean Six Sigma Approach*

**Donald E. Lighter, MD, MBA, FAAP**
Director, The Institute for Healthcare
Quality Research and Education
Knoxville, Tennessee

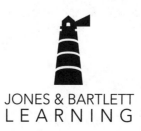

JONES & BARTLETT
LEARNING

*World Headquarters*
Jones & Bartlett Learning
5 Wall Street
Burlington, MA 01803
978-443-5000
info@jblearning.com
www.jblearning.com

Jones & Bartlett Learning books and products are available through most bookstores and online booksellers. To contact Jones & Bartlett Learning directly, call 800-832-0034, fax 978-443-8000, or visit our website, www.jblearning.com.

**Production Credits**

Publisher: Michael Brown
Managing Editor: Maro Gartside
Editorial Assistant: Chloe Falivene
Production Assistant: Rebekah Linga
Senior Marketing Manager:
   Sophie Fleck Teague
Marketing Manager: Grace Richards
Composition: Cenveo Publisher Services
Cover Design: Scott Moden
Cover Image: © Molodec/ShutterStock, Inc.
Printing and Binding: Malloy, Inc.
Cover Printing: Malloy, Inc.

**Library of Congress Cataloging-in-Publication Data**
Lighter, Donald E.
  Basics of health care performance improvement : a lean Six Sigma approach / Donald Lighter.
    p. ; cm.
  Rev. ed. of: Quality management in health care / Donald E. Lighter and Douglas C. Fair. c2004.
  Includes bibliographical references and index.
  ISBN-13: 978-0-7637-7214-7 (pbk.)
  ISBN-10: 0-7637-7214-3 (pbk.)
  1. Medical care--Quality control. 2. Six sigma (Quality control standard) I. Lighter, Donald E. Quality management in health care. II. Title.
  [DNLM: 1. Quality Assurance, Health Care--organization & administration--United States. 2. Quality Assurance, Health Care--methods--United States. 3. Quality Indicators, Health Care--organization & administration--United States. 4. Total Quality Management--methods--United States. W 84.4 AA1]
  RA399.A1L54 2013
  362.1068--dc23
                              2011027800

6048

Printed in the United States of America
15  14  13  12  11        10  9  8  7  6  5  4  3  2  1

# Dedication

As with all my work, I dedicate this book to my faithful wife and life companion, Sally, and the wonderful family that she has helped create over the years.

# Contents

**Preface** ...................................... ix

**Chapter 1**  **Why Is Performance Improvement
the "Big New Thing"?** .......................1
Background ..................................... 5
Improving the Quality of Care ................. 8
Patient Safety–A Specific Quality Goal .......... 10
Reducing Cost .............................. 14
Quality Frameworks .......................... 15
When will Quality Become "Job 1"? ............ 17
Discussion Questions ......................... 18
References ................................. 19

**Chapter 2**  **Define Phase Tools** ........................ 21
Background ................................. 21
Project Charter ............................. 22
Voice of the Customer ........................ 26
    CAHPS Surveys and the Voice of the Customer ........ 30
    National CAHPS Benchmarking Database ............. 31
    Other Methods of Listening to the Voice
        of the Customer ............................ 32
Kano Model ................................ 35
    Procedure for Kano Model process ................... 37
    Tips and tricks .................................. 38
Stakeholder Analysis ......................... 39
    Procedure for stakeholder analysis and diagram ........ 41
    Tips and tricks .................................. 41
Process Mapping ............................ 41
    Procedure for creating a process flowchart ........... 42
    Tips and tricks .................................. 43

SIPOC Process Map  . . . . . . . . . . . . . . . . . . . . . . . . . . . 44
    Procedure for SIPOC process map  . . . . . . . . . . . . . . . . . . 44
    Tips and tricks  . . . . . . . . . . . . . . . . . . . . . . . . . . . . . . . . . 45
Brainstorming, Brainwriting, and Nominal
    Group Technique  . . . . . . . . . . . . . . . . . . . . . . . . . . . 47
    Procedure for brainstorming  . . . . . . . . . . . . . . . . . . . . . . . 47
    Variants–brainwriting and nominal group
        technique (NGT)  . . . . . . . . . . . . . . . . . . . . . . . . . . . 48
    Multivoting  . . . . . . . . . . . . . . . . . . . . . . . . . . . . . . . . . . . . 49
    Affinity diagrams  . . . . . . . . . . . . . . . . . . . . . . . . . . . . . . . 51
Critical-To-Quality (CTQ) Analysis  . . . . . . . . . . . . . 53
    Procedure for creating a CTQ tree  . . . . . . . . . . . . . . . . . 54
Completion of the Define Phase  . . . . . . . . . . . . . . . . . 55
Discussion Questions  . . . . . . . . . . . . . . . . . . . . . . . . . . 56
References  . . . . . . . . . . . . . . . . . . . . . . . . . . . . . . . . . . . 57

**Chapter 3**    **Measure Phase Tools**  . . . . . . . . . . . . . . . . . . . . . . . **59**
The Essence of the Measure Phase  . . . . . . . . . . . . . . . 59
Measure Phase Tools  . . . . . . . . . . . . . . . . . . . . . . . . . . 61
    Process Maps  . . . . . . . . . . . . . . . . . . . . . . . . . . . . . . . . . . 61
    Performance Evaluation and Review Technique
        (PERT) Chart . . . . . . . . . . . . . . . . . . . . . . . . . . . . . . . 62
    Deployment Flowchart  . . . . . . . . . . . . . . . . . . . . . . . . . . 69
    Prioritization Matrix  . . . . . . . . . . . . . . . . . . . . . . . . . . . . 72
    Process Cycle Efficiency (Value Added Ratio)  . . . . . . . . . 76
Time Value Analysis (TVA)  . . . . . . . . . . . . . . . . . . . . 79
    Pareto Charts  . . . . . . . . . . . . . . . . . . . . . . . . . . . . . . . . . 80
    Run Charts  . . . . . . . . . . . . . . . . . . . . . . . . . . . . . . . . . . . 83
    Control Charts  . . . . . . . . . . . . . . . . . . . . . . . . . . . . . . . . . 88
    Failure Mode and Effects Criticality
        Analysis (FMECA)  . . . . . . . . . . . . . . . . . . . . . . . . . . . 95
Deliverables in the Measure Phase  . . . . . . . . . . . . . . 100
    Data Collection and Analysis Plan  . . . . . . . . . . . . . . . . 100
    Measurement System Analysis  . . . . . . . . . . . . . . . . . . . 103
Baseline Performance—
    Calculating Process Sigma  . . . . . . . . . . . . . . . . . . . . 105
Finishing the Measure Phase  . . . . . . . . . . . . . . . . . . . 107
Further Reading  . . . . . . . . . . . . . . . . . . . . . . . . . . . . . 108
Discussion Questions  . . . . . . . . . . . . . . . . . . . . . . . . . 108

**Chapter 4**   **Analyze Phase Tools** ........................ **111**
The Essence of the Analyze Phase .............. 111
Elements of the Analyze Phase ................. 112
Root Cause Analysis (RCA) ....................... 113
Cause and Effect (C&E) Diagram ................. 117
Statistical Methods of Establishing Relationships ...... 120
Pearson Correlation Coefficient .................... 121
Hypothesis Testing ............................. 125
Confidence Interval ............................. 131
Analysis of Variance (ANOVA) ................. 133
Regression Analysis ............................ 138
Brainstorming in the Analyze Phase ............. 141
Deliverables of the Analyze Phase .............. 141
Discussion Questions .......................... 143
References ................................... 144

**Chapter 5**   **Improve Phase Tools** ........................ **145**
The Essence of the Improve Phase .............. 145
Elements of the Improve Phase ................. 146
Framework for the Improve Phase .............. 146
Traditional Improvement Tools ................ 148
Change Management ........................... 148
Project Plan ................................... 150
Failure Mode and Effects Analysis (FMEA) ........... 151
Kaizen ........................................ 152
6S ............................................ 158
Prioritization Matrix ........................... 163
Deployment Flowchart .......................... 163
Pilot Testing .................................. 165
Six Sigma Tools ............................... 168
Completing the Improve Phase ................. 173
Discussion Questions .......................... 173
References ................................... 174

**Chapter 6**   **Control Phase Tools** ........................ **175**
The Essence of the Control Phase .............. 175
Elements of the Control Phase ................. 176
Framework for the Control Phase .............. 176
Control Phase Tools .......................... 181
Flowcharts .................................... 181
Standardization and Institutionalization
of Process Changes .......................... 183
Training Plans and Programs ..................... 191

Monitoring Plans ............................... 195
Poka Yoke ...................................... 196
Audit Plans .................................... 199
Control Charts ................................. 201
Process Sigma Level ............................ 209
Control Phase Deliverables ................... 210
Discussion Questions ......................... 210
Other Resources .............................. 211
Risk Adjustment .............................. 212
References ................................... 212

**Chapter 7    LSS Case Studies in Health Care ............. 215**
Miami Baptist Hospital ....................... 216
Pocono Medical Center (PMC),
    East Stroudsburg, PA ...................... 218
Nebraska Medical Center Peggy D. Cowdery
    Patient Care Center ...................... 221
Radia, Inc. .................................. 224
Providence St. Joseph Medical Center (PSJMC),
    Burbank, CA .............................. 229
North Shore-Long Island Jewish Health System,
    New York City ............................ 234
Discussion Questions ......................... 240
References ................................... 241

**Chapter 8    DMAIC in an Era of Reform ................ 243**
Trends in Healthcare Reform .................. 243
New Financial and Quality Realities .......... 250
Financial Models ............................. 252
Quality Reporting and Improvement ............ 257
Health Information Technology (HIT) .......... 260
Role of DMAIC as a Quality
    Improvement Strategy ..................... 261
Discussion Questions ......................... 262
References ................................... 263

**Appendix    Quality Measures for Accountable Care
    Organizations ......................... 265**

**Glossary    DMAIC Terms and Definitions ............. 283**

**Index ..................................... 317**

# Preface

Lean Six Sigma has become a rallying cry in the healthcare industry around the world as a way of achieving the value proposition of high quality at low cost. However, as discussed in Chapter 1, we in the industry have a long way to go. We're still allowing errors to creep into our work, even as society is becoming more demanding and less tolerant of those errors. The United States has lost the claim of being "the best healthcare system in the world," as statistics on mortality rates and other key health metrics have shown, but many practitioners like to claim that we're still number one in access to expensive technology. If that were a valid criterion for quality care, then our healthcare quality statistics should far exceed those of other nations. We do, however, exceed the performance of nations similar to ours in one measure: cost per capita. As shown in Chapter 1, the cost per person for health care in the United States far surpasses that of every other country in the world. Clearly, the situation must change.

The Six Sigma and lean production systems were created by engineers at Motorola nearly four decades ago and engineers at Toyota over five decades ago, respectively. Each had merit in its niche, and each paradigm was responsible for lifting entire segments of the United States' and Japanese economies out of stagnation and declining performance. Now the healthcare industry around the world has begun to increasingly adopt these approaches to revitalize healthcare performance as well. Healthcare reform passed in 2010 in the United States (the Patient Protection and Affordable Care Act), and that act has placed even more emphasis on the need for the industry to change. Incentives are aligning with performance (i.e., quality metrics) rather than just volume, while at the same time payments for services will soon be capped or begin to decline. The Center for Medicare and Medicaid Services (CMS) has instituted policies that eliminate payments for complications caused by "never events," (e.g., retained foreign bodies after surgery and pressure ulcers sustained during medical care) which places increased pressure on hospitals in particular to eliminate errors. Additionally, new payment approaches like bundled payments for specific medical procedures will begin to pressure providers to reduce costs and improve efficiency. Thus, Lean Six Sigma (LSS), a combination approach that has worked well in other sectors of the economy, appears to be a natural solution for these new market contingencies.

As I set out to write a basic quality improvement (QI) text, it occurred to me that the basics of QI had changed. Most high performing organizations had already adopted LSS, and those that are aspiring to higher performance are in the process of implementing this more advanced framework. So, rather than a traditional textbook on quality improvement, I determined that this iteration of the "basics" would involve an approach that would lead to even higher performance. This book is flexible in its usage and application. Students in health administration programs will find this book provides an excellent foundation in the fundamentals of QI. At the same time, the book is designed as a practical reference to help senior executives understand the basics of the LSS approach, as well as to support teams as they begin to implement LSS in their organizations. DMAIC (Define-Measure-Analyze-Improve-Control) is the acronym that LSS practitioners use to summarize the approach, and the book is organized to explain each of these steps in great depth for LSS teams and leaders to use for training and for support during a DMAIC initiative. The prior book in this series, *Advanced Principles and Methods of Performance Improvement in Health Care*, can serve as a companion to this text, as it puts LSS into context with other performance improvement models and takes a deep dive into some of the concepts. The goal of this book is to provide the depth in LSS that can take organizations to higher operational levels that will ensure sustainability as health consumers change the marketplace to value-based purchasing.

Any book of this type requires effort and advice from many people and sources to ensure precision and accuracy (see Chapter 3), and I would like to thank a number of people, including my family for their support during the writing of the text and Dr. Adam Campbell who helped review the statistics discussions. I also have the privilege of teaching these topics in the Physicians' Executive MBA program at the University of Tennessee in Knoxville, and discussion with students and other professors in the program have been particularly valuable for making this text a reality. Finally, my coworkers in Lean Six Sigma, Roger Noble and Diane Jenkins, have helped shape important parts of the book as well.

Donald E. Lighter, MD, MBA, FAAP

# CHAPTER 1

# Why Is Performance Improvement the "Big New Thing"?

*"Change is not necessary. Survival is not mandatory."*

—W. Edwards Deming

Americans are annoyed. The United States spends the greatest amount for health care of any developed country, but quality of health care measured by statistics like infant mortality rate lags far behind other countries. Consider, for example, the following statistics from the 2008 Commonwealth Fund's National Scorecard on US Health System Performance:[1]

- The US infant mortality rate at 6.8 per 1,000 live births exceeds that of Japan, Iceland, Sweden, Norway, Finland, Denmark, and Canada (**Figure 1-1**).
- Healthcare costs as a percent of GDP are higher in the US than in any other industrialized country (**Figure 1-2**).
- People who experience problems affording medical bills increased from 34% in 2005 to 41% in 2007 according to the Commonwealth Fund Biennial Health Insurance Survey (**Figure 1-3**).
- Recently, a Medicare beneficiary complained to a Florida health plan that an oncologist was demanding payment from the patient for the

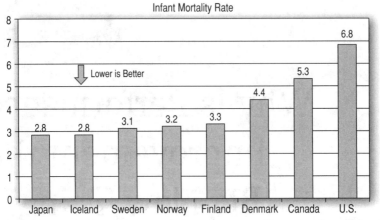

Data from: McDorman M, Mathews T, Recent Trends in Infant Mortality in the United States, NCHS Data Brief, No. 9, October, 2008, accessed at http://www.cdc.gov/nchs/data/databriefs/db09.pdf

**FIGURE 1-1**  Infant mortality rate comparison 2004

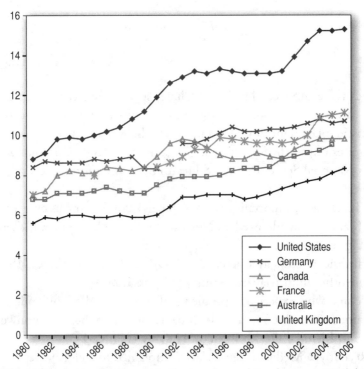

Data from: Organization for Economic Cooperation and Development, 2007 data

**FIGURE 1-2**  Comparison of healthcare costs as a percent of GDP

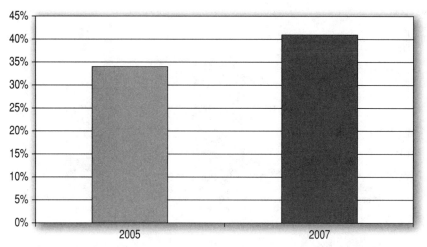

Data from: Doty M, Collins S, Rustgi S, Kriss J, Seeing Red: The Growing Burden of Medical Bills and Debt Faced by U.S. Families, The Commonwealth Fund Issue Brief, 42: August 20, 2008, accessed at http://www.commonwealthfund.org/Content/Publications/Issue-Briefs/2008/Aug/Seeing-Red--The-Growing-Burden-of-Medical-Bills-and-Debt-Faced-by-U-S--Families.aspx

**FIGURE 1-3** Percent of adults (ages 19–64) with any medical bill problem or outstanding debt

portion of a chemotherapy regimen not covered by Medicare. The oncologist refused to initiate therapy until this "copayment" (the part that is not covered by Medicare) was remitted. Some of these therapeutic medications can have a copayment of several thousand dollars. The elderly man reported that he was in the process of remortgaging his house so that he could afford the treatment, saying "If I lose the house, I can live on the street. That's better than losing my life."[2]

- Despite increased spending in Medicare and Medicaid, ethnic disparities persist in a number of basic healthcare measures, such as access to a primary care physician (**Figure 1-4**).

- In addition to the high cost and variable quality of the US healthcare system, only 64% of US physicians are satisfied or very satisfied with the system in which they work, among the lower percentages in the industrialized comparison group (**Figure 1-5**).

These issues dominate the US healthcare market in the early 21st century. Although a large proportion of the population is covered by health insurance, coverage is spotty, incomplete, and the tens of millions of people

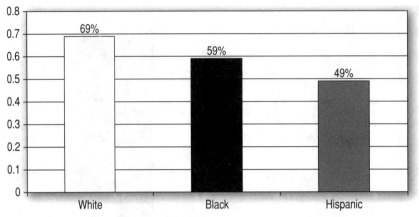

Data from: Medical Expenditure Panel Survey, 2011

**FIGURE 1-4** Variation in access to primary care physician by ethnic group 2005

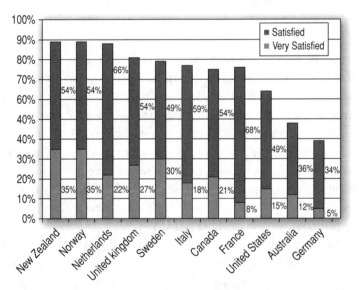

Data from: 2009 Commonwealth Fund International Health Policy Survey of Primary Care Physicians

**FIGURE 1-5** Percent of primary care physicians satisfied or very satisfied with medical practice 2009

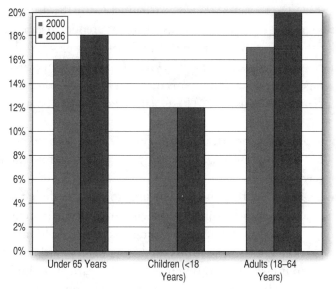

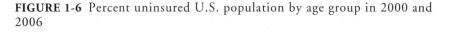

Data from: Analysis of Current Population Survey, March 1995–2007

**FIGURE 1-6** Percent uninsured U.S. population by age group in 2000 and 2006

who are not covered are at risk of a catastrophic event ruining their lives (**Figure 1-6**). After a generation of cost cutting showed little effect on cost or quality, healthcare delivery systems in the US and other industrialized countries around the world have begun to focus on the tenets of performance improvement. The expected benefits of this new direction subsume three areas: 1) quality of care, 2) patient safety, and 3) cost.

## BACKGROUND

The 1970s and 1980s saw the start of the wave of managed care, which ostensibly was to help ensure appropriate care in appropriate settings with appropriate follow up. Unfortunately, the first three decades of managed care consisted mainly of "managed cost," i.e., finding ways of decreasing the utilization of health services mainly by placing barriers in the way of providers (doctors, nurses, and other practitioners) being able to request and obtain care for patients.[3] Practices like prior authorization, concurrent review, and retroactive denials using rules that sometimes bordered on the arcane combined to thwart access to care by increasing the difficulty faced by practitioners and their patients in assuring that rendered care would be paid for by the insurance companies. In the 1990s a new wrinkle arose, consumer driven health care (CDHC). CDHC plans do not provide "first dollar coverage," i.e., the first amounts incurred for services are paid by the patient, rather than the insurer. These plans have two key characteristics:

- A high deductible health insurance policy, often with deductibles of $2,500–$5,000, that must be paid by the patient before the insurer starts paying.
- A savings account that the patient uses to pay the deductible. The savings account can be filled by the employer or the patient may be required to pay into the account through payroll deductions. In some cases, amounts in these accounts can be carried forward into the next year, without taxation, creating incentives for patients to limit care to only those medical services that are most likely to be valuable.

Unfortunately, high deductible plans may discourage individuals from getting preventive screenings like mammograms, Pap smears, and colorectal screening, in an effort to avoid depleting the savings account. Equally unfortunate are the consequences of ignoring these important screenings – later diagnosis of treatable conditions leading to more expensive treatment and less favorable outcomes of otherwise curable diseases. In short, people who are at financial risk for healthcare services simply do not see the value in many preventive care services.

Additionally, because of the gross disparities in care, as well as the financial inequities in the system, public sentiment has increasingly turned to advocating a complete overhaul of the healthcare delivery system. In a 2009 survey by the Commonwealth Fund, 15% of US physicians stated that the system needs to be completely rebuilt, and 67% opined that the system needs fundamental change.[4] As of this writing, the parameters of the new healthcare industry plan are being hotly debated in both Congressional and public forums, but it is clear that some type of change is in the offing.

Less well known, however, is the change in reimbursement policies by the Centers for Medicare and Medicaid Services (CMS), which is slowly reshaping the system even more than the reforms being reviewed in the political arena. CMS has begun using quality scores to determine levels of payment for health plans. These "Star Ratings" are presently based on three

**Table 1-1** Components of the health plan Star Ratings report

| | Stands for: | Explanation |
|---|---|---|
| **HEDIS** | Health Effectiveness Data Information Set | • Clinical and administrative measures for health plans, hospitals, and ambulatory settings<br>• Operational definitions based on ICD codes<br>• Derived from health plan transaction data and chart reviews |
| **CAHPS** | Consumer Assessment of Health Performance Survey | • Survey of consumers of health care<br>• Versions for health plans, hospitals, ambulatory settings (e.g., physician offices)<br>• CMS contractors conduct surveys of health plan members<br>• Determines satisfaction with health plan member services, primary care physician services, specialist services |
| **HOS** | Health Outcomes Survey | • Tracks a cohort of health plan members over two years<br>• Initial "paper" survey completed by health plan member, followed up with telephone survey two years later to determine difference in health status<br>• Scores derived from consumer perception of health status improvement |

Data from: Kaiser Family Foundation, What's In the Stars? Quality Ratings of Medicare Advantage Plans 2010, Issue Brief, December, 2009, accessed at http://www.kff.org/medicare/upload/8025.pdf

components: HEDIS scores, CAHPS scores, and HOS scores (**Table 1-1**), as well as Medicare administrative (primarily complaint) data. Performance in these three measurement systems is combined according to a statistical formula, and the resulting score is compared with other health plans to rank the plans according to their aggregate performance on the measures. The rankings are used to determine rates for payments of the health plans that are then reflected in member benefits (lower payments lead to fewer included benefits), provider payments (particularly incentives), and in some cases, health plan viability.

In this way, CMS intends to incentivize health plans to push the quality agenda to its providers and members. Although this approach is unproven to date, aligning incentives to desired behaviors is expected to produce desired results; however, the "law of unintended consequences" will likely surface other effects, as well. For example, if health plans withdraw from Medicare because of the financial changes, then a smaller number of health plans will assume responsibility for larger numbers of members, creating "mega-plans" that may be more difficult to control through negotiations and incentives. As this new system of quality incentives unfolds, these unintended outcomes must be continually reviewed. As the incentive program is promulgated through Medicare, it will gradually morph into similar programs in state Medicaid plans, as well as many commercial plans.

## IMPROVING THE QUALITY OF CARE

The healthcare industry has responded to this renewed emphasis on quality of care in a number of ways specific to the sector. Providers (i.e., physicians, nurses, therapists, and others who deliver medical care to patients) have adopted approaches from industrial engineering to improve the effectiveness and efficiency of care. Health plans have initiated efforts to prod members and providers into adhering to guidelines based on evidence from medical literature and clinical experts. Patients and providers alike find themselves in an ideal position if they are motivated to encourage and adopt preventive care practices, since the most highly subsidized metrics are those that encourage preventive care and wellness. The fact that the entire healthcare system is refocusing on quality does not necessarily ensure success, however. Incentives for each of the many participants in the system (**Figure 1-7**) overlap, but do not align. For example, consider these conflicts:

- **Patients** want unfettered access to the most advanced and safest care possible for themselves and their families. If a provider wants to do a test or implement a treatment, then it should be allowed, regardless of the evidence of efficacy. The advent of Internet sites on health care and direct-to-consumer advertising by pharmaceutical companies have raised public awareness of diagnostic and therapeutic modalities, but do not always include information on appropriateness. Most practitioners have had the experience of patients bringing printouts from the Internet on a clinical condition or treatment and demanding tests or medications that may not be appropriate. The patient's position is understandable, as no one would want to suffer deleterious health

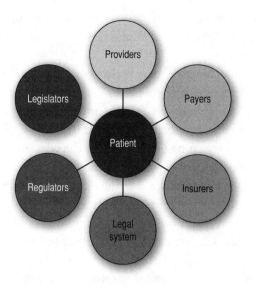

**FIGURE 1-7** The health care accountability circle

consequences because of lack of access to care or failure of a provider to consider all possible alternatives. This shrinkage of the medical information gap between providers and patients has increased the demand for services, sometimes inappropriately.

- **Physicians** want to do their best to ensure patients have the best and most advanced care, but many also are driven by the need to run a business, as well as to generate enough of a profit to make it worth eight years of education and three or more years of postgraduate residency and fellowship training. Theories of physician pricing behavior suggest that physicians maintain target incomes based on a number of factors, including specialty and site of practice.[5] Thus, pricing by physicians for many years was based on the amount of marginal revenue needed to meet that target. Now, however, the fees paid to physicians are mostly set by governmental or commercial insurers, and so the only factor in the revenue equation (Revenue = Volume x Price) is the volume of services. Thus, for physicians to meet these targets, they must increase volume. On the other hand, physicians are trained as scientists who are motivated to apply science and technology to the care of patients, which has led to some of the extraordinary advances in the past 50 years. The motivation to use these techniques to improve care is compelling for physicians who want to improve the lives of patients and practice the science of medicine. Physicians' incentives are thus complex, but critical to the cost and quality of care.

- **Payers** may be lumped into three groups: 1) insurers, who serve as the intermediaries for payments; 2) employers, who offer health insurance to employees as a benefit; and 3) government entities that pay for the health care for the poor and the elderly, either directly or through insurance companies similar to the way employers use insurers as intermediaries. The cost of health care has increased dramatically in the past five decades, putting extraordinary financial pressure on payers and consuming more resources that could be devoted to a business's core competency. For example, one of the factors that brought mighty General Motors to bankruptcy was the cost of health care for employees and retirees.[6] Payers have become focused on containing healthcare costs, and that effort has translated into realigned incentives for employee wellness programs and limits on payments for care, i.e., cost containment programs enforced through insurers.

Only when incentives among all of these participants become aligned will the system finally achieve the value proposition – i.e., the highest possible quality at the lowest possible cost. Achieving this alignment is perhaps the greatest challenge of healthcare reform. Simply changing the payment system to reward outcomes will not be sufficient: indeed, providers must also adopt approaches that enhance care and reduce errors, and consumers must take an active interest in their health by employing preventive services and healthy lifestyles.

## PATIENT SAFETY—A SPECIFIC QUALITY GOAL

Improving the quality of care is a rather general concept, but it translates into one important goal, that of patient safety. Healthcare providers for decades averred that healthcare services were safe, although not necessarily without risk. When the landmark book by the Institute of Medicine, *To Err Is Human: Building a Safer Health Care System,*[7] estimated that 98,000 preventable deaths in the US occur annually due to medical errors, the reaction by healthcare providers followed the classic Kübler-Ross model, starting with denial and finally ending with acceptance after several years of public debate. The actual number has become less important than the need to eliminate medical errors and preventable morbidity. Patient safety has become the new mantra of the industry, and a number of important initiatives have emanated from this guiding principle.

- **The Joint Commission (TJC)** has implemented a number of important programs for provider organizations, including:
  - **National Patient Safety Goals (NPSGs)**—a program started in 2002 to serve as a method for organizations to focus on patient safety. The Patient Safety Advisory Group, consisting of physicians, nurses, pharmacists, and other health professionals, reviews the medical literature each year to determine opportunities for improving patient safety and then translate those opportunities into specific measures that can direct initiatives for improvement.
  - **"Do not use" list**—recognizing the issue of misinterpretation of abbreviations in medication orders, TJC initiated the "do not use" list in 2005, which included such shortcuts as "cc" and "μg". The goal of implementing this list is to eliminate a common source of error in medication ordering. Seventy professional organizations participated in a summit in 2004 to ratify the list and add it to TJC standards.
  - **Infection control**—TJC has partnered with a number of organizations, including the Society for Healthcare Epidemiology of America (SHEA, www.shea-online.org), to develop guidelines for reducing hospital acquired infections (HAIs). HAIs are a leading cause of morbidity and mortality in medical settings, and the infectious organisms have become increasingly resistant to available antimicrobials; thus, HAI prevention has become a primary strategy for providers. The *Compendium of Strategies to Prevent Healthcare-Associated Infections in Acute Care Hospitals*, available for free download on SHEA's Web site, has become a seminal publication in these efforts.[8]
  - **Speak up**—TJC created this award-winning program to empower patients to become engaged in their care and to add another set of eyes to the care team. The program's name is an acronym for:
    - **S**peak up if you have questions or concerns. If you still don't understand, ask again. It's your body and you have a right to know.

- **P**ay attention to the care you get. Always make sure you are getting the right treatments and medicines by the right healthcare professionals. Don't assume anything.
- **E**ducate yourself about your illness. Learn about the medical tests you get and your treatment plan.
- **A**sk a trusted family member or friend to be your advocate (advisor or supporter).
- **K**now what medicines you take and why you take them. Medicine errors are the most common healthcare mistakes.
- **U**se a hospital, clinic, surgery center, or other type of healthcare organization that has been carefully checked out. For example, The Joint Commission visits hospitals to see if they are meeting The Joint Commission's quality standards.
- **P**articipate in all decisions about your treatment. You are the center of the healthcare team.
- **Universal protocol**—starting in 2004, TJC began monitoring hospitals and ambulatory surgery facilities for implementation of the Universal Protocol for Preventing Wrong Site, Wrong Procedure, Wrong Person Surgery. Created to address the continuing occurrence of wrong site, wrong procedure, and wrong person surgery, the Universal Protocol strengthened requirements from the 2003 NPSGs and required three steps in the preoperative period:
  - Preprocedure verification process to validate the patient's identity and procedure
  - Marking the procedure site to avoid operating on the wrong location
  - Performing a time-out before the procedure to revalidate the patient's information
- The **Agency for Healthcare Research and Quality (AHRQ)**, a division of the US Department of Health and Human Services, has become a treasure trove of patient safety information that is provided at no charge to the public. A few of these programs include:
  - **Online journals**—these journals provide the latest information on research into preventing errors and improving patient safety
  - **Patient Safety Network**—a Web site with articles and a newsletter to identify risks and provide tools for mitigation (http://www.psnet.ahrq.gov/)

- **Patient Safety Primers**—a Web site with several basic texts and articles on patient safety and other improvement topics (http://www.psnet.ahrq.gov/primerHome.aspx)
- **Morbidity and Mortality Rounds on the Web**—cases involving medical errors or "good catches" for demonstrating patient safety principles (http://webmm.ahrq.gov/)
- **Tips for consumers and patients**—a Web site with information for consumers that can be used by providers for producing handouts and other patient education resources (http://www.ahrq.gov/consumer/5steps.htm)
- **TeamSTEPPS™ National Training Network**—resources for implementing a Crew Resource Management program (http://teamstepps.ahrq.gov/)
- **Patient Safety Organization (PSO) resources**—PSOs were authorized by the Patient Safety and Quality Improvement Act of 2005 to improve the quality and safety of US healthcare delivery by encouraging clinicians and healthcare organizations to voluntarily report and share quality and patient safety information without fear of legal discovery (http://www.pso.ahrq.gov/)
- The **Institute for Healthcare Improvement (IHI)** supports patient safety on its Web site with discussions, tools, and other resources.[9] The IHI has sponsored numerous collaborative sessions that examine patient safety issues and develop interventions to create a safer healthcare system.
- Many "no blame" safety reporting Web sites have arisen, such as that sponsored for the state of New Jersey by the state Department of Health and Senior Services.[10] These sites were developed to encourage reporting of patient safety problems that have occurred in practice in a way that does not involve blame assessment, with the goal of obtaining enough data to analyze for designing patient safety interventions based on error prevention and process improvement.

The compelling need to improve patient safety has placed increasing emphasis on quality improvement, which uses tools like root cause analysis, failure mode and effects criticality analysis, and sets Six Sigma limits to reduce errors to very low levels.[11] The Six Sigma approach has become more prevalent in the healthcare industry over the past several years, and evidence indicates that the approach is effective, if deployed correctly.

Carolyn Pexton of GE Healthcare reviewed several Six Sigma initiatives at several healthcare organizations and found success when the following factors were present:[12]

- Strong leadership involvement and support
- Techniques to promote culture change and break down silos
- Selecting the "best and brightest" for Six Sigma leadership
- Project-based training and mentoring for an adequate number of Green Belts, Black Belts, and Master Black Belts
- Selecting and scoping projects to achieve financial and quality results
- Measurable objectives aligned with organizational goals
- Clear roles and responsibilities
- Over-communicating by a factor of 1,000
- Attention to the Control Phase to maintain results
- Project tracking and reporting capabilities
- Accountability and recognizing achievements

These diverse approaches—patient safety tools and interventions, Six Sigma, and institutional initiatives—are directed at the issue of patient safety, a problem that has finally achieved "top of mind" status in the healthcare industry. Society is demanding safer care, but at the same time pressure is mounting to reduce the cost of care as well, which is the third major issue facing the industry.

## REDUCING COST

Although the Six Sigma philosophy fits best with the need to improve patient safety by reducing errors, it also can apply to improving efficiency. On the other hand, the lean process management approach pioneered by Toyota in the 1950s has been effectively applied to improving efficiency in healthcare organizations. Many healthcare institutions have adopted some semblance of the Toyota Production System (TPS) to reduce nonvalue-added work and associated costs. The TPS includes a number of tools that can be applied to process improvement and management, all targeted at reducing unnecessary effort and what is termed "muda" (waste) in the lean process management paradigm. Notably, TPS and Six Sigma approaches use many of the same tools, which will be described in later chapters.

Six Sigma has provided remarkable cost savings in a number of industries, however. General Electric, one of the pioneers in use of Six Sigma, demonstrated the efficacy of the approach in cost cutting.[13] Other companies have shown similar results, and some healthcare organizations have also produced cost savings by improving the quality of their operations.[14] These results are part of the reason that lean and Six Sigma have become such important philosophies in quality management in the healthcare industry.

## QUALITY FRAMEWORKS

As we begin to delve into the tools used by quality improvement (QI) professionals, it is important to establish a framework for use of these tools. A traditional QI framework established by Shewhart decades ago is "Plan-Do-Check-Act," often abbreviated PDCA. As indicated in **Figure 1-8**, this cycle follows a prescribed sequence of steps that is repeated iteratively until a desired goal is achieved. Each step of the sequence has a particular set of associated tasks:

- **Plan**—evaluation of a quality problem and development of a solution to the problem
- **Do**—implement the solution over a predetermined time period
- **Check**—measure the effects of the intervention using metrics defined during the Plan Phase
- **Act**—determine if the intervention was successful and set up control mechanisms to perpetuate the new process

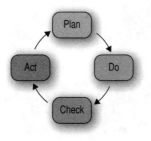

FIGURE 1-8 Plan-Do-Check-Act Cycle

Once the cycle has completed it may be repeated to continually refine solutions to quality issues. This approach has been used successfully in many industries for many years, and actually served as the basis for the Six Sigma approach developed by Bill Smith and Mikel Harry at Motorola in the 1980s.

Six Sigma started as the brainchild of Smith and Harry in response to serious quality problems at Motorola. They were given the job of bypassing the typically incremental gains of the company's quality system and developing a program that would set higher goals and achieve objectives more quickly. Building on PDCA, they proposed another framework—MAIC—which evolved to DMAIC, which stands for Define-Measure-Analyze-Improve-Control. This framework, as shown in **Figure 1-9**, extended PDCA with more advanced statistical tools to create a measurement-oriented system that ensured improvements that could be demonstrated with objective metrics. We will use the DMAIC framework to examine the tools available to the quality professional throughout this book.

The similarities between these two approaches are important to note since DMAIC was a natural progression from PDCA; however, DMAIC emphasizes some important characteristics of quality that have become standard in health care, e.g., the concepts of understanding a problem through use of data and statistical analysis prior to intervening and of ensuring that any gains achieved through an intervention are sustained by putting appropriate quality assurance methods in place. These concepts are easily understood in health care, since they serve as the basis for treatment

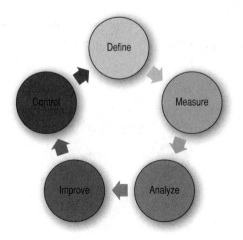

**FIGURE 1-9** Define-Measure-Analyze-Improve-Control

and diagnostic modalities. For example, when a practitioner encounters a patient with hypertension, diagnostic procedures are performed and analyzed to determine the underlying cause of the condition, and then specific therapies are applied to remedy the situation. Once a therapeutic combination has demonstrated efficacy, the practitioner uses the information to implement programs to maintain the gains through maintenance medications, lifestyle changes, and other approaches. Thus, the diagnostic and therapeutic framework used in treating patients closely parallels that of DMAIC, making the paradigm particularly resonant with healthcare workers.

## WHEN WILL QUALITY BECOME "JOB 1"?

A popular Ford automobile commercial in the 1980s featured employees from a variety of sites in a Ford Motors facility stating: "At Ford, quality is Job 1."[15] Although the US automotive industry suffered immensely during the economic downturn in 2008, Ford actually remained afloat without external assistance, and emerged in a stronger position after the recession ended. This resilience is in part due to shrewd financial management, but it also can be ascribed to this renewed emphasis on quality. Similarly, the importance of quality measurement, improvement, and reporting has grown immensely in recent years. Hospitals have become particularly scrutinized, and the Centers for Medicare and Medicaid Services have made hospital quality information available on the Web.[16] This Web site allows comparison of hospital quality data across several hospitals and is searchable in several ways, like zip code, city name, state, or county, and then stratifies the data by clinical condition or surgical procedure, if desired. Other institutions are also featured on CMS Web sites:

- Nursing Homes—www.medicare.gov/NHCompare
- Home Health Agencies—www.medicare.gov/HHCompare
- Dialysis Facilities—www.medicare.gov/Dialysis

Additionally, Medicare health maintenance organizations (HMOs) and Part D drug plans (PDPs) are ranked on separate Web sites:

- Medicare Advantage plans (HMOs)—www.medicare.gov/MPPF
- Part D plans—www.medicare.gov/MPDPF

In addition to these federally sponsored sites, other organizations have also created Web sites for comparing healthcare entities. A few examples include:

- North Carolina Hospital Quality Performance Report (http://www .nchospitalquality.org/)—a site sponsored by the North Carolina Hospital Association that compares overall performance of hospitals in the state for several clinical conditions (e.g., heart attack, heart failure, pneumonia, and surgical care) using publicly available data.
- The Joint Commission (www.qualitycheck.org)—a Web site sponsored by the largest US accreditation organization with data from accreditation reports for every institution that they review.
- The Leapfrog Group (www.leapfroggroup.org)—a consortium of US industrial giants and other businesses, The Leapfrog Group has worked for many years to improve the effectiveness and efficiency of the healthcare industry. The organization now reports on multiple measures through a voluntary reporting system for a variety of clinical conditions. The database is searchable by a number of location factors, such as city, state, or zip, and the results may be displayed graphically or in numeric format.
- HealthGrades (www.healthgrades.com)—this Web site provides reports on physicians and other healthcare providers by locality. These reports pull data from a variety of public sources and assemble a report of each physician, hospital, or nursing home. Although these reports are costly, they provide a reasonably comprehensive view of each provider.

Consumers now have several ways to review and evaluate quality data about providers and payers, and the public reporting of this information will create a drive for healthcare organizations to improve performance that should help make quality become "Job 1." The application of quality improvement tools will ensure that quality professionals will have an important part to play in the healthcare delivery system for decades to come.

## DISCUSSION QUESTIONS

1. Discuss the evolution of managed care payment systems in societal efforts to control healthcare costs and improve quality. How has the federal government been involved?

2. In what ways has the healthcare industry responded to society's concerns about the quality and safety of health care? Discuss the approaches taken by each sector of the industry.

3. What programs have organizations like The Joint Commission, the Institute for Healthcare Improvement, and the Agency for Health Research and Quality formulated to improve quality and safety in health care?

4. Explain the use of "no blame" safety reporting programs in identifying and remediating quality of care issues.

5. How does quality relate to cost? Can improvements in quality and safety reduce costs? Why or why not?

6. What is the PDCA cycle? How does it relate to improvement of healthcare quality?

7. What is DMAIC? How does it relate to improvement of healthcare quality?

8. What will stimulate the healthcare industry to make quality "Job 1"?

# REFERENCES

1. The Commonwealth Fund. (July 2008). *The Commonwealth Fund Commission on a High Performance Health System, Why not the best? Results from the National Scorecard on U.S. Health System Performance, 2008.* Retrieved from http://www.commonwealthfund.org/Content/Publications/Fund-Reports/2008/Jul/Why-Not-the-Best--Results-from-the-National-Scorecard-on-U-S--Health-System-Performance--2008.aspx.

2. Lighter, D. (December 2009). [Personal Communication].

3. Mains, D.A., Coustasse, A., & Lykens K. (2004). Physician incentives: Managed care and ethics. *The Internet Journal of Law, Healthcare, and Ethics*, 2(1). Retrieved from http://www.ispub.com/journal/the_internet_journal_of_law_healthcare_and_ethics/volume_2_number_1_30/article/physician_incentives_managed_care_and_ethics.html.

4. The Commonwealth Fund. (2009). *Commonwealth Fund International Health Policy Survey of Primary Care Physicians.* Retrieved from http://www.commonwealthfund.org/Content/Surveys/2009/Nov/2009-Commonwealth-Fund-International-Health-Policy-Survey.aspx.

5. Farley, P.J. (1986). Theories of the price and quantity of physician services. A synthesis and critique. *Journal of Health Economics*, Dec;5(4), 315–33.

6. McCracken, J., Langley, M., & Stoll, J. (2009, March 30). Bankruptcy leads possible plans for GM, Chrysler. *The Wall Street Journal.* Retrieved from http://online.wsj.com/article/SB123841609048669495.html.

7. Kohn, L.T., Corrigan J.M., & Donaldson, M.S. (Eds.). (2000). *To err is human: Building a safer health system.* Washington, DC: National Academy Press.

8. The Society for Healthcare Epidemiology in America. (2009). *Compendium of strategies to prevent healthcare-associated infections in acute care hospitals.* Retrieved from http://www.shea-online.org/about/compendium.cfm.

9. Institute for Healthcare Improvement. *Patient safety.* Retrieved from http://www.ihi.org/IHI/Topics/PatientSafety/SafetyGeneral/.

10. State of New Jersey. (2009). *Patient safety.* Retrieved from http://www.state.nj.us/health/ps/.

11. Pexton, C. (2005). One piece of the patient safety puzzle: Advantages of the Six Sigma approach. *Patient Safety & Quality Health Care,* January/February 2005. Retrieved from http://www.psqh.com/janfeb05/sixsigma.html.

12. Pexton, C. (2009). *Measuring Six Sigma results in health care.* Retrieved from http://healthcare.isixsigma.com/library/content/c040623a.asp#Carolyn.

13. Waxer, C. (2010). *Six Sigma costs and savings: The financial benefits of implementing Six Sigma at your company can be significant.* Retrieved from http://www.isixsigma.com/library/content/c020729a.asp.

14. Koning, H., Verver, J., van den Heuvel, J., Bisgaard, S. & Does, R. (2006). Lean Six Sigma in health care. *Journal of Healthcare Quality,* 28(2):4-11. Retrieved from http://www.nahq.org/journal/ce/article.html?article_id=250.

15. Paton, S.M. (2000). No small change: making quality job 1, again. *Quality Digest.* Retrieved from http://www.qualitydigest.com/sept01/html/ford.html.

16. United States Department of Health and Human Services. (2011). *Hospital compare.* Retrieved from http://www.hospitalcompare.hhs.gov.

# CHAPTER 2

# Define Phase Tools

*"A goal without a plan is just a wish."*

—Antoine de Saint-Exupery

*"In preparing for battle I have always found that plans are useless, but planning is indispensable."*

—General Dwight D. Eisenhower

*"An expert is one who avoids the small errors while sweeping on to the grand fallacy."*

—Anonymous

## BACKGROUND

Every improvement project must start with a thorough understanding of the quality issue to be improved. A common error at this stage is to assume that one person's perception of a problem is correct, without examining supporting data or at least other perceptions that can provide more insight into an issue. The Define Phase of the improvement cycle avoids such errors through a structured problem analysis that examines an issue and develops a process map to unambiguously communicate the elements of a process that are working well and those that are not working very well. One key to an effective improvement effort is a clear understanding of the process, as well as the goals and objectives for change. The deliverables from the Define Phase help communicate process issues and improvement goals in a manner that should be understandable by all stakeholders.

Define Phase tools that will be discussed in this chapter include the following:

- Project charter
- Voice of the Customer
- Kano model
- Stakeholder analysis
- Process mapping, including SIPOC process map
- Brainstorming and its variants
- Multivoting and list reduction
- Affinity diagram
- Critical-to-quality (CTQ) analysis

The goal of applying these tools is to produce several key deliverables, including:

- Fully trained team
- Customers identified
- High impact characteristics (CTQs) defined
- Team charter
- Process mapped
- Adequate budget
- Senior leadership support

The key to ensuring a highly effective outcome for the project is inherent in those deliverables.

# PROJECT CHARTER

It is useful to think of the charter as a contract between leaders and the project team. Created at the outset of the project, the purposes of the project charter are numerous:

- To clearly state the purpose and goals of the project
- To provide background on the reason(s) for the project

- To ensure alignment of project and team goals with organizational priorities
- To identify resources available and constraints for the project
- To delineate deliverables and define success

The project charter is the document that the team leader uses continuously to keep the team focused on the task and expected outcomes. Other stakeholders usually receive an executive summary of the project to serve as a reminder of the project's importance, timeline, and deliverables. Senior managers can refer to the project charter when evaluating resource allocation decisions to ensure that the return from the project is justified by the expected outcome.

Project charters vary substantially in structure and content, but in general the document should include the elements listed in **Table 2-1** and include the following:

- Background and purpose
  - What prompted the interest in the project?
  - Where is the project positioned in the organization's priorities?
  - Which organizational leaders and/or departments are most interested and invested in the outcome?
  - Which systems in the organization have been malfunctioning and to what extent?
  - What is the underlying reason for the project (e.g., cost containment, patient safety, member satisfaction, etc.)?
  - Over what period of time has the issue developed?
  - How quickly does the organization need a solution?

**Table 2-1** Project charter contents

| Charter element | Description |
| --- | --- |
| **Background and purpose** | • Description of the process or issue to be addressed and its importance to the business<br>• Problems with the current process—what motivated the project? |
| **Mission statement** | • Succinct statement of the project purpose and goals that includes the purpose and direction for the team<br>• Links to organizational mission statement should be evident |

**Table 2-1** Project charter contents (*continued*)

| Charter element | Description |
|---|---|
| Scope | • Boundaries and limitations |
| | • Project outcomes—what goals must the project achieve? |
| | • Project milestones—timeline of steps (sometimes called "gates") that will be achieved during the project |
| | • Deliverables—what reports, measures, processes, products, or services will the project deliver when complete? |
| | • Cost estimates—budgetary limits for the project, including staff time and costs for other resources |
| | • Organizational interfaces—departments or workgroups expected to be affected by the project |
| | • Other stakeholders affected by the project |
| | • Urgency/priority of the project |
| | • Source of team empowerment (e.g., Senior Vice President of Health Services) and allowed functions (e.g., review and execute contracts) |
| Team composition and roles | • List of functional areas, skills, levels of expertise, and external stakeholders who need to be represented on the team, usually divided into core team members and extended team members |
| | • In some cases, specific names may be included in the list |
| | • Roles for each of the team members (e.g., leader, subject matter expert, recorder, etc.) |
| Operational framework | • Special environmental factors (e.g., team work locations, software, computers, etc.) |
| | • Accountability—who on the team is accountable for which parts of the project? |
| | • Decision-making processes—methods for making and reporting decisions (e.g., majority vote, super majority, weighted voting) |
| | • Conflict resolution rules and procedures—final authority for any conflicts that arise |
| | • Process improvement tools and procedures |
| | • Procedures for changing team members and/or leaders |
| Performance measures | • Measures of team performance, such as deadlines for deliverables |
| | • In-process metrics to determine level of success for team, such as results of pilot test, process efficiency measures |
| | • Outcome measures for project (e.g., goals achieved) |
| Support requirements | Any other support needed, like consultants, special measurement systems, facilities, outside vendors |

- Mission statement
  - Succinctly describe the mission of this project; mission statements should be two or three sentences at most and capture the essence of the goals and objectives of the effort
  - Relationship of the project mission to the organizational mission statement
- Scope
  - Departments and divisions affected by the project
  - Economic and budgetary limits for project activities and recommendations
  - Business and work processes affected by the proposed project
- Team composition and framework
  - Core team members—those team members who will participate throughout the project
  - Additional team members—those team members whose expertise may be needed from time to time, but not continuously throughout the project
  - Consultants—specialized staff or external resource people who may be needed for specific issues
  - Support staff—administrative staff who facilitate the team's work, such as taking and preparing meeting notes, arranging for meeting space, etc.
- Operational framework—the improvement or planning paradigm to be used by the team for executing the project; for example, the team may use a company-specific improvement model or the DMAIC model or perhaps a lean model
- Performance measures—a list of all measures that will be used to assess the project, including:
  - Structural—infrastructure elements required for a project or the underlying process to be improved; these measures can involve equipment, staffing, capital investment, physical facilities, or information systems
  - Process—in-process metrics usually include milestones or "gates" that indicate the project is proceeding according to the planned schedule
  - Outcome—these measures vary widely by project, but usually include an implementation plan for the new process, as well as a "scorecard" of measures to assess the process going forward

- Support requirements—any other support requirements not previously mentioned in the charter, such as particular senior leader team sponsorship

In some cases, the executive(s) that commission the project may provide the charter, but if not, then the leadership team for the project should ensure that a charter is created and confirmed by the executive(s) before starting to work. A project charter template is included as **Figure 2-1** and at the online resource center for this book.

## VOICE OF THE CUSTOMER

The best place to start with any project is a thorough understanding of the customer in as many dimensions as possible. Customer characteristics, like basic demographics (name, address, contact information) constitute some of the key data elements of any project, but other traits, such as ethnicity, gender, and age, may also help in project planning as a means of tailoring a service or product to a particular population. For example, if a team wanted to develop a program to improve blood pressure control in a population that included a subset of Mandarin Chinese people, then surveys and educational information may need to be adapted to accommodate unique language and cultural needs. This information is used to develop methods of obtaining the **"Voice of the Customer" (VOC)**, which involves the process of capturing feedback from customers to better understand their requirements. The VOC process is not a one-time project, but rather systematic development of a "listening and learning" culture that obliges all employees to collect formal and informal customer feedback to drive continuous improvement of the organization's services and products.

The VOC process needs to capture both stated and unstated customer requirements using tools such as those in **Table 2-2**. Perhaps the most widely used method of gaining insight into customer requirements in health care is the standardized survey. Companies like Press Ganey (http://www.pressganey.com) and  NRC Picker (http://www.nrcpicker.com) have developed validated questionnaires for healthcare organizations to use to query customers regarding issues like promptness of service, facility cleanliness, staff friendliness, time spent with the doctor, and other satisfaction issues. These services have substantial associated costs, and so many smaller providers (e.g., medical office practices) are unable to afford to survey patients in this manner.

| Project Charter for | | | | |
|---|---|---|---|---|

| Project Name: | Project Number: | Prepared by: (Project Manager) | Date Submitted: |
|---|---|---|---|
| Customer: | Department: | Contact: | Project Type: |

| Project Start Date: | Project End Date: | Milestone 1 | Milestone 2 | Milestone 3 | Milestone 4 | Milestone 5 | Milestone 6 |
|---|---|---|---|---|---|---|---|

**Background and Mission:**

**Scope:**

Business Case Summary:

Business Goals:

Project Objectives:

Deliverables:

Beneficiaries:

Key Requirements:

**Resources:**

| Core Team: | Name | Department | Weekly Time Commitment | Start Date | End Date | Comment |
|---|---|---|---|---|---|---|
| | | | | | | |
| | | | | | | |
| | | | | | | |
| | | | | | | |
| | | | | | | |
| | | | | | | |
| | | | | | | |
| | | | | | | |
| | | | | | | |
| | | | | | | |

| Adjunct Team Members: | | | | | | |
|---|---|---|---|---|---|---|
| | | | | | | |
| | | | | | | |
| | | | | | | |
| | | | | | | |
| | | | | | | |
| | | | | | | |

**FIGURE 2-1** Project charter template

| Other Human Resourceces: | | | | | | |
|---|---|---|---|---|---|---|
| IT | | | | | | |
| Support Staff | | | | | | |
| Consultant | | | | | | |
| Ancillary Resources: | Description | Number or Degree | Weekly Time Commitment | Start Date | End Date | Comment |
| Travel | | | | | | |
| Supplies | | | | | | |
| Software | | | | | | |
| Hardware | | | | | | |
| Training | | | | | | |
| Other | | | | | | |

| Risk Assessment (With and Without Project): |
|---|
| Risk if Project Done-risks Associated With Project |
| |
| Risks if Project not Done-business and Other Risks of Status Quo |
| |
| Constraints and Boundaries |
| |

| Budget | | | | | | | | | |
|---|---|---|---|---|---|---|---|---|---|
| | Description | Staff | Consultants | IT | Travel | Supplies | Hardware | Software | Training | Totals |
| | | | | | | | | | | $ - |
| | | | | | | | | | | $ - |
| | | | . | | | | | | | $ - |
| | | | | | | | | | | $ - |
| | | | | | | | | | | $ - |
| | | | | | | | | | | $ - |
| | | | | | | | | | | $ - |
| | | | | | | | | | | $ - |
| | | | | | | | | | | $ - |
| | | | | | | | | | | $ - |
| | | | | | | | | | | $ - |
| Total | | $ - | $ - | $ - | $ - | $ - | $ - | $ - | $ - | $ - |

| Summary |
|---|
| |

Sign Off:

| | | |
|---|---|---|
| | | . |
| Project Manager | Supervisor | Executive Sponsor |

**FIGURE 2-1** Project charter template *(continued)*

**Table 2-2** Voice of the Customer data collection methods

|  | Formal | Informal |
|---|---|---|
| **Stated** | Individual structured interviews | Individual open interviews |
|  | Standardized surveys | "Quicky" questionnaires |
|  | Focus groups | Spontaneous group sessions |
|  | Formal proposal specifications | Customer inquiries and requests |
|  | Complaint logs | Customer complaints to staff |
| **Unstated** | Structured observation of customer behavior | Staff observations of customer behavior |
|  | Warranty data and product returns |  |
|  | Medical-legal actions |  |

Fortunately, the Agency for Healthcare Research and Quality (AHRQ, http://www.ahrq.gov) has funded development and validation of a number of survey tools known as the Consumer Assessment of Healthcare Providers and Systems (CAHPS) surveys. Since these surveys were developed through federal grants, the surveys and comparison datasets are available on the AHRQ Web site at no charge. The CAHPS Consortium, a panel of survey experts, has led the development of several instruments since the mid-1990s and continues to build and support a wide-ranging and growing family of standardized surveys that poll consumers and patients on their experiences with health care and include such issues as provider communication skills and access to care.

## Detail: The CAHPS Consortium

The CAHPS Consortium consists of federal agencies and private research organizations. The federal agencies include one of the primary funders of the project beginning with the first CAHPS survey for health plans, the Centers for Medicare & Medicaid Services (CMS). Other federal agencies involved in CAHPS include the Centers for Disease Control and Prevention and the National Institute for Disability and Rehabilitation Research. Private researchers are awarded grants for their participation in the program and include experts in survey development, quality assessment and improvement, and reporting, such as Harvard Medical School, Research Triangle Institute, and RAND. For the second phase (CAHPS II), AHRQ funded five-year cooperative agreements with the American Institutes for Research, Harvard Medical School, and RAND, and for the most recent phase (CAHPS III), the Consortium added the Yale School of Public Health and RAND. The Agency also has engaged Westat to support the work of the Consortium and the CAHPS User Network, as well as managing the National CAHPS Benchmarking Database.

CAHPS surveys include instruments for assessing the quality of care in both ambulatory and institutional settings, and each survey package includes the survey questionnaire, administration protocols, analysis and reporting guidelines programs, and guidance in reporting results.

## CAHPS Surveys and the Voice of the Customer

The first CAHPS survey was developed to measure consumer satisfaction with health plans, and this instrument has become the standard by which health plans are measured and, in recent years, classified for incentive programs. The CAHPS Health Plan Survey is used by commercial, Medicaid, State Children's Health Insurance Program (SCHIP), and Medicare plans representing more than 120 million enrollees. Consumers can view results of the surveys on the CMS Web site (https://www.cahps.ahrq.gov/CAHPSIDB/Public/About.aspx), and the CAHPS survey is one of the components behind the Medicare Star Ratings report (http://www.cms.gov/PrescriptionDrugCovGenIn/06_PerformanceData.asp) that ranks health plans on Health Effectiveness Data Information Set (HEDIS), CAHPS, and Health Outcomes Survey (HOS) performance. Additionally, the National Committee for Quality Assurance (NCQA) incorporates CAHPS results into both its health plan performance reports as well as its health plan accreditation process.

The Consortium also developed surveys during the second phase of CAHPS that assess consumer experience in ambulatory settings, such as physician offices, managed behavioral healthcare organizations, dental plans, and tribal clinics. The standardized, validated approach to data acquisition and reporting make them invaluable for any organization to measure the voice of the customer in these specific settings. Additionally, the ambulatory care survey[1] includes optional supplemental items that may be added to specific instruments without changing the validity of the instrument.

CAHPS surveys include instruments tailored for patient satisfaction measurement in other healthcare facilities, such as hospitals, nursing homes, and dialysis centers. The CAHPS Hospital Survey, often referred to as H-CAHPS or Hospital CAHPS, focuses on adult inpatient satisfaction with hospital care and services. Hospitals across the country have adopted the survey for measuring inpatient satisfaction and voluntarily report their data to CMS for inclusion in the CAHPS database used for benchmarking and comparisons. Another CAHPS survey has been fielded for use in hemodialysis centers for patients with end stage renal disease, and a nursing home survey is nearly ready for distribution.[2]

AHRQ supports the surveys through a variety of no-cost services, which include the CAHPS User Network and the National CAHPS Benchmarking Database. The CAHPS User Network helps users with technical questions and allows users to interact with each other and CAHPS researchers. The User Network provides the following resources:

- **Free technical assistance**—users can pose questions via a toll-free number (800-492-9261) and an e-mail address (cahps1@ahrq.gov)
- **A comprehensive CAHPS Web site** (www.cahps.ahrq.gov), which houses the following:
  - CAHPS Survey and Reporting Kits—questionnaires, reporting measures, administration protocols, analysis programs, and instructions for using the CAHPS products
  - New and upcoming CAHPS products
  - Resources to support implementation of a survey project, public reporting of survey results, use of CAHPS surveys to improve quality, and translation of CAHPS surveys to other languages
  - Searchable FAQs and bibliography
  - Materials and other information developed for CAHPS events, webcasts, and national user group meetings
  - Resources designed to support users in identifying and networking with other organizations that are doing similar or related work
- **Newsletter**—*The CAHPS Connection* newsletter[3] keeps users informed about new programs, events, and survey changes

## National CAHPS Benchmarking Database

Not only does the CAHPS survey provide a validated resource for gathering patient satisfaction in a number of settings, but the system includes a benchmarking database to compare an organization with others that are similar. The database incorporates data from commercial and Medicaid plans that has been collected for over a decade. CAHPS program sponsors can obtain reports that compare survey results to database benchmarks, access data from individual surveys, and receive customized reports for a fee. The database has become an important source for research into consumer evaluations of healthcare quality in each of the survey domains.

## Other Methods of Listening to the Voice of the Customer

Survey methods are widely used in health care to hear the VOC. However, astute healthcare organizations have learned a number of other ways to understand customer requirements, including:

- Formal customer listening methods
  - Complaints/appeals/grievances
  - Customer comments and questions
  - Focus groups
  - Retention/referral analyses
  - Kano model
- Informal customer listening methods
  - Short informal surveys
  - Community networking
  - Web site

One of the most useful ways of determining customer dissatisfaction is by analyzing customer complaints to determine system issues and trends. For example, if customers register a large number of complaints about the noise level on a hospital unit, the staff should evaluate the sources of the noise and work to eliminate them. In some cases, the trend in number of complaints also can be helpful in discerning targets for intervention. Many healthcare organizations monitor their complaint logs, often by capturing complaints in a database and categorizing them for analysis. Tracking these complaint categories can help quality improvement staff to determine upward trends in certain issues that, although they may not have reached a critical threshold, may represent opportunities for improvement. Complaints in provider organizations are usually handled through a formal process such as that described in **Example 2-1**, but complaints in payer organizations are managed somewhat differently. Because state and federal oversight agencies consider customer complaints to be important indicators of health plan quality and access to care, a system of managing these problems has evolved that generally involves three levels of severity:

1. **Complaint**—a health plan member calls the member service line to complain about a service, provider, or to request assistance receiving a service that has been denied. If the member service coordinator can resolve the issue at that encounter, the complaint is considered closed.

2. **Grievance**—if the member service coordinator is unable to resolve the complaint, then the complaint is usually converted to a grievance, which escalates to health plan staff for further review to determine if the complaint can be decided to the member's satisfaction. If the result is not acceptable to the member, the next step is an appeal.

3. **Appeal**—if the health plan has not resolved the grievance to the member's satisfaction, then the issue is referred to an outside arbiter, such as an administrative law judge, for final adjudication. This level generally represents the final step in the process.

Health plans track the appeals and grievance process to find opportunities for improvement, as well as indications of the effectiveness of its utilization management programs.

---

## Example 2-1 Complaint log analysis

Perfect Sat Hospital maintains a customer complaint log that allows entry of patient complaints either directly by patients via the Web site or by any staff member who receives a complaint from a customer. As the data are entered into the log, each complaint is categorized into one of five domains: 1) staff, 2) facilities, 3) dietary/nutrition services, 4) administrative functions (e.g., billing, collections, etc.), and 5) physicians. The staff tracks the *rate* of complaints per 1,000 patient days by graphing them on a control chart, adding a new point each month. When a point indicates a special cause, the staff immediately launches a Root Cause Analysis (RCA) to determine the underlying cause. The staff also evaluates the trend of complaints to determine if an upward (unfavorable) or downward (favorable) trend is present. If an upward trend is detected, the staff investigates the underlying causes using either a RCA or a Failure Modes and Effects Analysis (FMEA).

---

In addition to surveys and formal complaint processes like that in Example 2-1, quality oriented organizations also develop methods of capturing customer comments and complaints that may be expressed in more informal ways. For example, many organizations will encourage employees to record and report comments made by customers during informal encounters during their daily work. For example, (true story) an employee at a hospital observed a four-year-old sibling of another child skipping down the hallway singing "we're gonna sue you!" She reported the observation to the risk managers at the hospital who intervened with the parents and helped defuse the situation. In addition to mitigating obvious risks, these informal observations may also identify some other opportunities for improvement, such as cleaning services or dietary department performance.

Focus groups are typically used to get more in-depth customer views regarding a concept, product, or service. These facilitated sessions are led by a moderator who leads a group of participants through a discussion on a particular topic that follows a plan with questions, prompts, tasks, and exercises. The success of a focus group depends on the moderator, who must generate interest in the subject, involve the entire group, direct the discussion loosely enough to allow for digressions that might provide more information about the topic, and avoid directing the group in a way that reflects the sponsor's expectations. The focus group is often most effective in gaining insights from group interactions, as well as individual contributions to the discussion. For example, if a new product is being reviewed, the group might be given a prototype to examine both individually and as a group. After group members have worked with the prototype, they can come together and discuss their reactions. Outcomes and deliverables from a focus group include notes and transcripts of the sessions, sometimes in audio or video format. The facilitator or sponsor usually creates a report summarizing the purpose of the study, a description of the procedures, detailed findings, and significant themes that emerged within and between focus group sessions. Focus groups are usually fairly inexpensive, but in the hands of an unskilled facilitator, the information gained from a session may be misleading. As with any survey technique, data from a focus group can be distorted by poor memory, unwillingness to be truthful, and subject selection bias. Moderators must have the requisite skills to conduct effective group sessions and manage the vagaries of group behavior.

Customer retention and willingness to refer are often included as part of customer satisfaction surveys; for example, the requisite questions are included in CAHPS surveys. Analysis of this data is important to determine the likelihood of customers returning to the organization. New customers almost always require some investment in marketing, advertising, and other outreach activities, while returning customers do not require that level of investment. Thus, retaining current customers should be a high priority for any organization, and efforts to improve service quality and cost are the most effective ways of achieving that goal. Additionally, customers who would refer their family and friends to the organization are also an important indicator of organizational quality and effectiveness, and these referred customers generally cost less to recruit. Finding the underlying reasons for loss of customers and unwillingness to refer helps identify opportunities for improving the organization's services.

Finally, many institutions have informal methods of getting information from customers, such as conducting their own short surveys of customer satisfaction. These short questionnaires usually focus on a specific aspect of service that one of the service units wishes to evaluate. For example, a patient care unit may wish to learn more about customer satisfaction with pain management, while the billing office may want to better understand complaints related to billing errors. Rather than change the process for the formal satisfaction survey, the unit may create and deploy a short survey, often consisting of just a few questions that are not on the standard patient satisfaction instrument. These short surveys focus on a specific problem and can help identify some specific improvement issues fairly quickly. Although they lack the rigor of a typical patient satisfaction survey, they are widely used to help staff understand and resolve specific quality problems.

In addition to the short surveys, organizational leaders and other employees may participate in community activities and collect comments from customers and other stakeholders for analysis as part of the VOC effort. Some other contemporary methods of gathering customer opinions and comments may involve interactive Web sites that provide the organization with unstructured but readily available customer data.

## KANO MODEL

Developed by Professor Noriaki Kano in the 1980s as a method of stimulating innovative product/service design, the Kano Model classifies customer preferences into five categories:

1. **Attractive quality**—These attributes relate to customer surprise and delight (i.e., they create high levels of customer satisfaction when achieved, but do not cause dissatisfaction when not achieved). These attributes are not usually expected (e.g., free valet parking at a hospital) and often are not verbalized by customers. W. Edwards Deming's statement, "The customer never asked Mr. Edison for a light bulb" provides an example of an unspoken feature. This dimension is often ignored, since it is usually difficult to ascertain.

2. **One-dimensional quality**—Quality attributes that result in satisfaction when fulfilled and dissatisfaction when not fulfilled are considered one-dimensional and are generally articulated by customers. Consider the dissatisfaction that travelers feel when a flight that is scheduled for 2:00 p.m. is delayed for two hours because of a mechanical problem on the airplane. These factors are sources of competitive advantage for high performing organizations.

3. **Must-be quality**—Customers view must-be attributes as inherent in the product or service, and when not present, customer dissatisfaction is quick and serious. For example, a patient scheduled for a visit with a specific doctor will not be any more or less satisfied when the doctor enters the room, but will be dissatisfied if another doctor appears instead. These attributes are also usually not communicated by customers, since they are part of a basic expectation of the service or product feature.

4. **Indifferent quality**—Indifferent quality refers to aspects that are neither good nor bad, and, consequently, they do not result in either customer satisfaction or customer dissatisfaction.

5. **Reverse quality**—In this domain, presence of an attribute creates dissatisfaction, and absence is associated with satisfaction, which emphasizes the fact that not all customers are alike. For example, some patients may like the use of advanced diagnostic instruments like PET scanners, while others may find the technology intimidating and unsatisfying.

A summary of these characteristics can be found in **Table 2-3**.

**Table 2-3** Kano model quality categories

| Quality category | Attribute present | | Attribute absent | |
|---|---|---|---|---|
| | Satisfaction | Dissatisfaction | Satisfaction | Dissatisfaction |
| Attractive | ⇑⇑ | ⇔ | ⇔ | ⇔ |
| One-dimensional | ⇑ | ⇓ | ⇓ | ⇑ |
| Must-be | ⇔ | ⇔ | ⇓⇓ | ⇑⇑ |
| Indifferent | ⇔ | ⇔ | ⇔ | ⇔ |
| Reverse | ⇓ | ⇑ | ⇑ | ⇓ |

## Procedure for Kano Model process

Kano model analysis really can be reduced to asking two basic questions about each attribute:

1. Rate your satisfaction if the product has this attribute?
2. Rate your satisfaction if the product did not have this attribute?

Responses to the questions should be one of the following:

- Very satisfied
- Satisfied
- Neutral (don't care)
- Dissatisfied
- Very dissatisfied

The procedure for conducting a Kano Model analysis involves the following:

1. Determine which product or service attributes are to be included in the analysis.
2. If the attribute is new or not well understood, consider writing a short summary of the attribute without adding judgmental language (e.g., we think this will improve the use of the product).
3. Determine the method of obtaining customer feedback. Surveys may be done in paper format, online via a Web site, through focus groups, or telephone.
4. Create the survey instrument using the questions and response levels above.
5. Field the survey and collect results.
6. Analyze the results using a Kano Model graph similar to **Figure 2-2** to determine if the attribute is one that produces sufficient customer satisfaction to warrant allocation of resources to ensuring the attribute's presence. Attributes that create customer delight generally receive more resources, while those that fall into the indifferent or reverse quality categories may be quickly eliminated.

The Kano Model helps prioritize specific product or service attributes so that the team can concentrate time and resources on those issues that will create the greatest traction with customers.

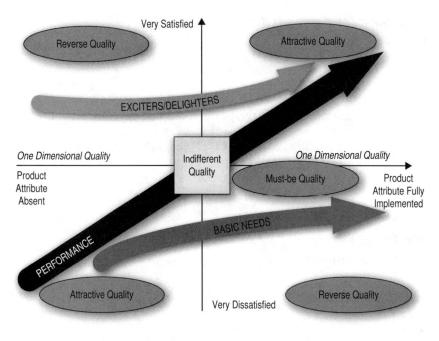

**FIGURE 2-2** Kano Model

## Tips and tricks

1. The team must try to quantify the attribute by extent of deployment. Using a five-point scale from "not deployed" to "fully deployed." The resulting value is then combined with the customer value from the survey to produce a point on the Kano Model graph.

2. The Kano Model graph demonstrates the three major areas of Attractive, One-Dimensional, and Must-be quality. Note that the Indifferent quality is represented by points clustered around the intersection of the x- and y-axes, and Reverse quality points would be reflected by a point that is very low on the customer satisfaction score, while Reverse quality points would be found in the lower right quadrant of the graph.

3. Basic attributes generally receive the "Neutral" response to Question 1 and the "Dissatisfied" response to Question 2. Exclusion of these attributes in the product may have a negative impact on the success of the product in the marketplace.

4. The Kano Model can be used in a number of circumstances other than just evaluation of product attributes. For example, customers may be surveyed about proposed attributes of a new product or service and a Kano Model graph can be created. In this type of analysis, the customer is presented with varying levels of the attribute in a product or service and asked the two questions. The ratings from the survey are then plotted as described previously.

5. Inclusion of performance or excitement attributes often requires a trade-off analysis against cost. Since customers frequently rate attributes or functionality as important, the first question may be rephrased, "How much extra would you be willing to pay to add or increase the amount of this attribute?" This information may be better to help a team prioritize new attributes or increases in existing attributes and begin to calculate a return on investment.

6. Neutral or "Don't Care" responses usually imply that the attribute will neither increase customer satisfaction nor motivate the customer to pay an increased price for the product. Although it is tempting to simply dismiss these attributes, they may in fact serve an essential purpose for the product and may not be summarily eliminated. For example, the preoperative stop that is now required for surgical procedures to verify patient identity and surgical details may not be something for which a patient may be willing to pay, but it serves a useful purpose in reducing errors.

The information obtained from the Kano Model analysis, specifically regarding performance and excitement attributes, provides valuable input for quality teams as well as for strategic planning and process improvement. Designing the analytic tools requires forethought and some skill, and the results can help clarify customer requirements for product and service offerings.

## STAKEHOLDER ANALYSIS

Fundamental change in a process requires buy-in and support from multiple sources, including executive leaders, senior managers, people in the department(s) being affected, suppliers, and customers. One of the first evaluations that a team will perform in preparing for a project is determining the important stakeholders. The team must consider everyone who might have an interest in the change and determine how they might react to the new process. A method of stratifying stakeholders in terms of importance to the project and influence on the outcome can be useful to anticipate how to manage expectations and which stakeholders will require greater attention. Additionally, an importance-influence matrix can graphically demonstrate who is most important to the project and who can be expected to exert influence to ensure project success. An example stakeholder matrix is shown in **Figure 2-3**.

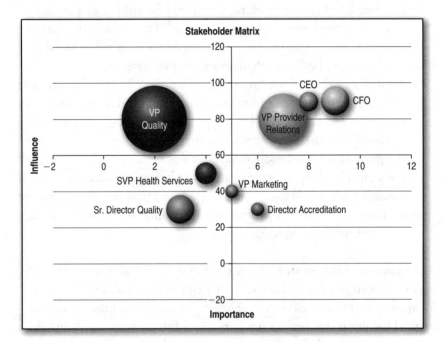

| Stakeholder | Importance | Influence | Magnitude |
|---|---|---|---|
| VP Quality | 80 | 80 | 6400 |
| Sr. Director Quality | 90 | 30 | 2700 |
| SVP Health Services | 40 | 50 | 2000 |
| VP Marketing | 30 | 40 | 1200 |
| Director Accreditation | 40 | 30 | 1200 |
| VP Provider Relations | 60 | 80 | 4800 |
| CEO | 20 | 90 | 1800 |
| CFO | 30 | 90 | 2700 |

**FIGURE 2-3** Stakeholder matrix

## Procedure for stakeholder analysis and diagram

1. Assemble team to determine stakeholders for project.
2. Create a list of potential stakeholders for the project.
3. Create a survey instrument that ranks each stakeholder on two dimensions: importance to the project and influence on the project.
4. Allow the team to rank each stakeholder on the two dimensions on a Likert scale (usually 1–9).
5. Enter the scores into a spreadsheet and average the rank scores for each stakeholder in each domain to create a table like that shown in Figure 2-3. Note the column labeled "Magnitude," which is the product of the two scores for importance and influence. The magnitude parameter determines the "size" of the bubble on the matrix.
6. Create a bubble chart like that shown in Figure 2-3 from the table by selecting the chart from the list of potential charts in Excel® using all three columns of data.

## Tips and tricks

1. If there is a chance that the stakeholder may have a negative influence on the project, the scale can be expanded to include negative numbers. For example, the Likert scale might range from -5 to +5, rather than 0 to 9.
2. The scale can be expanded (as shown in Figure 2-3) to any size (e.g., 0 to 100). Wider scales provide more choices and often avoid situations in which people may want to use 2.5 or 3.8 values.
3. Excel provides a method of placing text labels on each bubble as in Figure 2-3. The precise technique can be found in Excel Help in the topic "Add data labels to a chart" under the subtopic "Create a custom label entry."

# PROCESS MAPPING

Process mapping is a method of producing a workflow diagram that provides a graphic description of a process and related subprocesses. Process maps are ubiquitous tools for quality improvement teams to provide all stakeholders with a rapidly assimilated view of the process, as well as to hone in on specific steps that contribute to process variation or nonvalue added work. Process flowcharts are the result of the process mapping approach.

## Procedure for creating a process flowchart

1. Determine boundaries—establish the starting and ending points for the process

2. List the process steps—the level of detail depends on the use of the flow diagram; for example, if the flowchart is to be used to provide an overview for senior managers, less detail will be needed than if it is to be used by a process improvement team to find intervention points.

3. Put the steps in time sequence—the steps identified above should be placed in order based on when they occur in the process. Some may occur in parallel, while others will follow an ordered pattern. Many teams perform this task using a whiteboard or small notepaper, but it can just as easily be accomplished with a software program like Microsoft Visio®.

4. Draw the flowchart using appropriate symbols—flowcharting has a number of symbols to represent specific types of process steps, as shown in **Figure 2-4**. Although hundreds of flowchart symbols

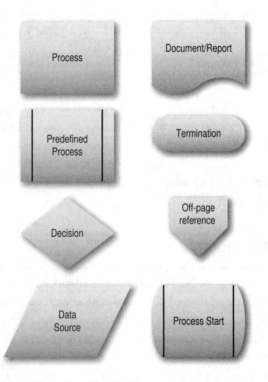

**FIGURE 2-4** Basic Flowchart Symbols

are available in software programs, the basic symbols in Figure 2-4 should suffice for most situations.

5. Obtain feedback on the flowchart from process owners and users—ensure that process owners and key process users agree with the flowchart before finalizing. It is often helpful to have a formal review process and sign off as a criterion for flowchart adoption.

6. Finalize the flowchart and distribute to appropriate stakeholders. The resulting flowchart should resemble the chart shown in **Figure 2-5**.

## Tips and tricks

1. Flowcharts benefit from both process user input and direct observation. Process users often have a concept of the process that may not conform to reality (i.e., because of constraints in the process, "workarounds" have become incorporated into the process flow that are now second nature to everyone involved). Thus, part of process mapping may involve a "walk through" of the process to try to detect variation that should be incorporated into the process map.

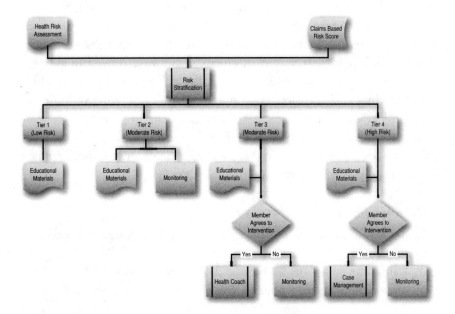

**FIGURE 2-5** Basic flowchart for diabetic care management program

2. The process map can be created individually or as a group. Although the group approach often takes more time, it usually offsets the time gaining feedback from stakeholders on a flowchart created by an individual.

3. Many teams create two flowcharts during this stage: one for the current state and one for the ideal state. The current state flowchart details the process in its present condition, complete with workarounds and other variation, while the ideal state flowchart provides the best possible process flow with variation and workarounds either removed or revised to accommodate ideal process flow.

# SIPOC PROCESS MAP

SIPOC is an acronym for **S**uppliers, **I**nputs, **P**rocess, **O**utput, and **C**ustomers and is used as a general description of the major process domains. In most cases, quality will be judged by the output of a process, but in process measures are used to gauge the efficiency and effectiveness of the process. Process outputs in a healthcare situation are usually services, such as a lab test or an imaging study or a diagnosis and subsequent treatment plan. In some cases, the quality of an output is difficult to assess, such as in a complex diagnostic situation when the output (diagnosis) is tentative and may take time to unfold. In many of these cases, output is measured indirectly by patient satisfaction with the outcome, rather than the accuracy of the outcome. In any case, efforts to improve output quality are directed at the preceding domains—suppliers, inputs, and process. Thus, understanding each of these components is important to any improvement project. An example of a SIPOC process map for performing a laboratory test is shown in **Figure 2-6**. The SIPOC process map is the high level overview of the process and allows a project planner to have a quick understanding of the major components of the process.

## Procedure for SIPOC process map

1. Identify suppliers, inputs, the basic process flow, outputs, and customers.

2. Using the template in **Figure 2-7** (created in Microsoft Visio), place each of the components into the appropriate column. Create a

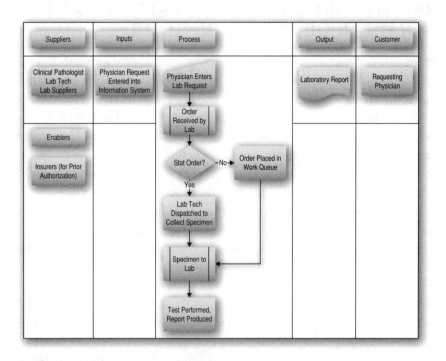

**FIGURE 2-6** SIPOC Process Map

high-level process flowchart for the process column using a flow-charting tool like Visio

3. Add details if needed, such as enablers. For example, if an insurer must authorize a test before it is performed, then the insurer could be considered an enabler under "suppliers."

## Tips and tricks

1. The process flowchart for the SIPOC process map does not usually have the same level of detail as a value stream map or working flow-chart. The SIPOC diagram is often paired with a traditional flow-chart that shows much more detail for in-depth process analysis.

2. Identifying the entries for each domain can usually be done through brainstorming with the well-formed team, but it also can be per-formed by a "walk around" observation of the process if ambiguities persist after the brainstorming session.

# BRAINSTORMING, BRAINWRITING, AND NOMINAL GROUP TECHNIQUE

Brainstorming and its variants, brainwriting and nominal group technique (NGT), are the most commonly used approaches to generating large numbers of ideas in a relatively short period of time. Nearly everyone has participated in a brainstorming session at one time or another, but it is likely that the level of preparation and planning that go into a successful brainstorming exercise may not be evident to participants. Brainstorming relies on group participation, and if a group is reticent or does not perform collaboratively, the other two approaches (brainwriting or NGT) may be preferable.

Brainstorming sessions strive for volumes of ideas, not necessarily high quality suggestions, and certainly not fully formed plans. Some brainstormed ideas fail to survive later scrutiny and analysis, and so everyone in the session needs to know that any idea should be brought to the fore, regardless of how outlandish it might sound at the time. Another important principle underlying brainstorming is the absolute need to eliminate any criticism of new ideas during the session. Participants must feel free to express ideas in a noncritical, supportive environment, or the likelihood of gaining any new insights will be severely limited. If the group is unable to perform in this manner, then brainwriting or NGT may be more effective approaches. Finally, members of the brainstorming team should feel free to build on others' ideas. In other words, if other team members can add to an idea that has already been presented, they should be encouraged to do so. The synergies achieved in this way can often be beneficial to the final product.

## Procedure for brainstorming

These sessions should be led by someone experienced in the technique. The leader must prepare for the session as follows:

- **Creation of a clear problem definition**—the problem should be stated as clearly as possible, with specific questions, (e.g., "How can we streamline laboratory flow to improve turnaround time?"). Brainstorming sessions benefit from the specificity of the problem statement, since participants can focus on specific ideas that are germane to the issue.
- **Summarize background**—the group will usually require a basic understanding of the problem; although participants are selected for their expertise in the issue, a summary of the fundamental issues surrounding the topic will help the group stay focused.

- **Select appropriate participants**—as noted previously, participants must be selected for their expertise and understanding of the issue to be discussed, and the three types of participants are usually managers, process owners, and customers of the process. In some cases, that group may include external customers, but usually the group consists of participants internal to the organization.
- **Prepare for the session**—ensure that all materials are prepared for the session and secure a location that facilitates the brainstorming process. Locations usually involve privacy and low levels of distractions, comfortable, and easily accessible for participants. Additionally, the leader should prepare for the situation in which group members lose focus and may require directed questions to consider in the process. For example, the leader may want to have questions ready like "What if a lab machine breaks? How should the process flow be modified?" or "How does the lab process flow accommodate emergencies?" The session leader should also ensure that all necessary supplies (timer, recording medium like a whiteboard or flipchart) are ready for the session.
- **Conduct the session**—the session leader must conduct the session according to the rules of the brainstorming process outlined previously. Participants must feel empowered to express themselves freely in a nonthreatening environment, and they must feel that every opinion is valued by the team. Conducting the session is straightforward:
  - Assemble the team for the session
  - Briefly describe the problem and the process and then discuss any questions about either topic
  - Identify a timekeeper and a scribe to take down ideas as they occur
  - Open the session for ideas. In most cases, setting a 10-minute time limit for each round of idea generation helps the group from becoming discouraged. Conduct as many 10-minute rounds as needed to exhaust new ideas
  - Tally the ideas for the group to review and for use in the next phase, which is often "list reduction," described later.

## Variants—brainwriting and nominal group technique (NGT)

Brainwriting is used when brainstorming is hampered by poor group dynamics, such as one or two dominant participants or a particularly difficult subject for discussion. Brainwriting is similar to Nominal Group Technique as a method of getting information from participants that may not be willing to share. The two techniques are similar in that participants write their ideas on a sheet of paper, rather than expressing them verbally in the group. The differences between the two approaches are listed in **Table 2-4**. One interesting variant of the brainwriting procedure is the use of diagrams instead of word descriptions for idea generation; thus, if a product design is the subject of the brainstorming session, participants might use figures or diagrams on the brainwriting sheets rather than describe the design in words.

## Multivoting

Once the brainstorming session is completed, the large number of ideas needs to be reduced to a manageable few, and two methods of performing this task are multivoting and affinity diagrams. This section discusses multivoting, which is preferable to a single up and down vote on each idea because it allows an idea that is favored by all team members, but perhaps not the top choice of any of the group, to rise to the top of the priority list. Additionally, the group can consider the complete list and any potential synergies during a multivoting exercise, which provides some context around the voting. Multivoting is useful as a group tool to narrow a long list of possibilities into a manageable, prioritized subset.

### Procedure for multivoting

Supply each team member with 10 slips of paper and a pencil, and have a whiteboard or flipchart to use for listing all of the options and recording votes. The facilitator should decide how many items can be on the final reduced list. In general, up to ten rounds of voting may be necessary to reach the final tally, but in most cases, only four or five rounds are usually needed to reduce a list.

1. Display the list of options and combine any obviously duplicated items.
2. Number the items on the list.
3. Working individually, each team member selects five items that he or she feels are most important and then ranks the choices in order of priority, with the first choice ranking highest. Each choice is written on a separate piece of paper, with the ranking underlined in the lower right corner.

**Table 2-4** Comparison of brainwriting and NGT

| | Brainwriting | NGT |
|---|---|---|
| **Participant factors** | • Some group members are substantially more vocal than others | • Some group members are substantially more vocal than others |
| | • Some group members think better in silence | • Some group members think better in silence |
| | • Some group members may not participate due to shyness or a feeling of intimidation | • Some group members may not participate due to shyness or a feeling of intimidation |
| | • All or some team members are new to the effort | • All or some team members are new to the effort |
| | • The issue is controversial or has created conflict within the organization | • The issue is controversial or has created conflict within the organization |
| **Procedure** | • Clearly state the subject of the brainstorming exercise and ensure that everyone understands the issue | • Clearly state the subject of the brainstorming exercise and ensure that everyone understands the issue |
| | • Hand out a sheet of paper to each participant | • Allow 5–10 minutes for each team member to individually write down ideas: as with any brainstorming exercise, volume is more important than content |
| | • Each team member begins writing ideas on the page, usually for 1–2 minutes | • Gather the group together and have each team member read one idea to the rest of the group; the facilitator records each idea on a flipchart or whiteboard: |
| | • At the end of the allotted time each person passes his/her sheet to the left |    o No discussion is allowed during the idea sharing |
| | • The next person reviews the prior person's work and adds new ideas to the sheet that enhance the initial idea or create a completely new subject |    o As the exercise proceeds, ideas may be generated spontaneously and not from the team members' lists |
| | • The cycle is repeated until the pages are filled and everyone has had the opportunity to see every sheet |    o Team members may "pass" his or her turn, and may then add an idea on a subsequent turn. |
| | • After a few cycles, have team members read the best idea from all ideas on the page in front of them |    o Set a time limit for the idea sharing and stop when the limit has been reached or when everyone has used all of their ideas |
| | • The facilitator lists these ideas on the flipchart or white board for further discussion and clarification | • The facilitator leads discussion of each idea, with the following rules: |
| | • The ideas are prioritized using list reduction techniques like multivoting, in which the ideas are ranked by group members in successive secret ballots until the list is narrowed to three or four choices |    o Originator of an idea must agree to wording changes |
| | |    o Ideas may be eliminated only by unanimous vote |
| | |    o Group discussion should focus on clarifying meaning, explaining the idea, or answering questions |
| | | • Ideas should be prioritized by the group using list reduction techniques like multivoting |

4. The facilitator collects the papers, shuffles them, and then records the tally on the flipchart or whiteboard. It is usually best to have a scribe record the individual rankings next to each item, and then to total the rankings for each selection.

5. If a decision is clear after any of the voting rounds, the process may stop. Otherwise, the facilitator conducts a brief discussion of the vote to review the voting data, emphasizing those items with large ranges in ranking (e.g., votes of both 1 and 5 ratings), to identify any apparent misunderstandings of each item. The discussion should not produce pressure on anyone in the group to change their vote.

---

## Example 2-2 Multivoting

A hospital team from three departments was tasked with developing a list of key customers to contact regarding a new service. The group brainstormed a list of 32 possible names, which exceeded the limit of funding that had been budgeted. To reduce the list to the budgeted number of 18 potential contacts, the group used multivoting to identify the top 18 candidates. A facilitator conducted the exercise according to the procedure outlined in the text, and during each voting round, group members selected six names to be prioritized. After the third round of voting, the list had been successfully narrowed to 18 names with rankings to guide the outreach efforts. The top ten customers had fairly homogeneous voting scores, but the remaining eight scores had a broader distribution of votes, indicating less agreement of the group on the priority scores for the last eight customers.

---

### Affinity diagrams

An affinity diagram graphically represents large numbers of ideas, opinions, or issues in a framework that demonstrates natural groupings. The diagram is created using the affinity process, which is conducted after brainstorming or one of its variants. This approach can be used as an alternative to multivoting, or it can be used before multivoting when a list of possibilities is so long that it is unmanageable. Two particular situations lend themselves to the affinity process:

- Sifting through large volumes of data to find patterns—for example to categorize a population of patients into demographic categories for further analysis of utilization patterns.
- Encouraging new patterns of thinking—the affinity process encourages people to think quickly and creatively, and so may help team members find new perspectives on a problem. The use of brainstorming as the first step in the affinity process ensures "out of the box" thinking if done properly.

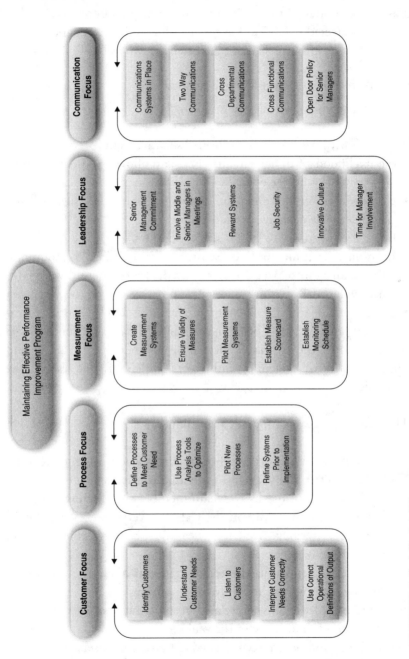

**FIGURE 2-7** Affinity Diagram

In general, if fewer than fifteen items of information have been identified as the target data set, the affinity process may be unnecessary. This process has been credited to Jiro Kawakita,[4] who published the approach in the 1960s, and so affinity diagrams are often known as KJs in his honor.

### Procedure for creating an affinity diagram

Underlying principles include the following:

- The affinity process is best performed silently. As the process unfolds, the likelihood of disagreements rises, and allowing discussion may divert attention to the overall task at hand.
- Constitute the group from people who understand the issues well and can discern the underlying relationships.
- Limit the group size to five or six participants.
- Encourage team members to use their initial reactions to groupings, rather than agonize over decisions. Gradual movement toward consensus will usually require an iterative process.
- Disagreements over classification are handled simply. If team members cannot agree on a position for one of the ideas within a single classification, the idea is duplicated on another sheet of paper and put under other categories until the team debriefs and resolves the conflict.

The affinity process is conducted as follows:

1. Conduct the brainstorming (or variant) session to generate a list of ideas. Write the ideas on individual pieces of paper (such as Post-it Notes) for use by the team members in the next step.
2. Post the ideas randomly on the wall for everyone to view. Avoid trying to "precategorize" the ideas by grouping them in any order.
3. Without conversation, the team then can place the ideas into related groupings in the following manner:
   - Find two ideas that seem related in some way and place them in a column off to one side of the wall.
   - Seek other ideas that seem related to those already selected and put aside, and then add them to that group.

- Repeat the process until all of the ideas have been used in some group.
- If some ideas are left as "mavericks," leave them in their own groups-of-one at this stage.

4. Create header cards for each group that capture the essential link among the ideas contained in the group. The header card may contain a short explanation of the grouping, as well as a simple title. Each header card is placed at the top of its respective group. Upon discussion, if two or more header cards seem to be related, they may be connected by a "superheader" card that is placed above those header cards. At this point, the group may engage in discussion to resolve some of the issues with ideas that have been placed in more than one group and the "mavericks."

5. Complete the exercise by drawing the affinity diagram like that in **Figure 2-7**.

### Tips and tricks

1. Ensure that the ideas are not in any particular order when starting the affinity process. If the notes are in some order at the start of the exercise, team members may be influenced in their thinking about the groupings.

2. Allow plenty of time for step three. Some affinity processes have occurred over several days. For example, the idea notes could be posted in a public place and arranged by a large group of people over several days.

3. Use markers to complete the idea notes to improve visibility from a distance. If the affinity process session is held in a large room, the information must be visible from a distance.

# CRITICAL-TO-QUALITY (CTQ) ANALYSIS

The methods for obtaining and organizing the Voice of the Customer represent the hallmarks of the Define Phase of a QI project. Once the surveys are completed or the brainstorming session has been conducted, however, a framework for understanding the VOC and converting it to actionable information is useful to provide direction to the project.

Critical-to-quality (CTQ) attributes are the key quantifiable customer requirements of a product or process that set performance standards or specification limits. CTQs help QI teams design initiatives that satisfy, or even delight, customers. One way of deriving CTQs from more general customer requirements is the CTQ tree.

## Procedure for creating a CTQ tree

1. **Identify key customer requirements** using the methods outlined previously (i.e., customer surveys, brainstorming [or its variants], affinity diagrams, etc.). These requirements may be as broad as necessary to adequately capture the customer's needs.

2. **Refine requirements using customer data or team experience**. For example, if customer service is an issue, the surveys may have identified telephone response time as an issue. Similar to a Root Cause Analysis, the team then begins to break down the issue into its component process steps to determine which step(s) are problematic. The team completes this phase when quantifiable requirements are reached. Thus, if telephone response time is the problem, then the team may discover that the three quantifiable issues are call pick up time (CTQ = 2 rings), time-to-human response (CTQ = 2 layers of answers to automated response system questions), and time on hold (CTQ = 20 seconds). Those three elements form the branches of the CTQ tree (**Figure 2-8**), which is created in the same manner as other decision trees.

3. **Confirm the final requirements with customers** to ensure that the analysis has yielded results that are likely to produce a benefit. The confirmation process may involve another survey targeted to these issues, informal conversations with key customers, or focus groups of a representative customer cohort.

The CTQ tree helps translate customer language into quantifiable requirements that can be used to develop improvement initiatives that have measurable outcomes. As such, the CTQ tree ensures that a comprehensive view of customer needs is used to identify key elements, and that an improvement team can transform relatively general needs into measurable interventions.

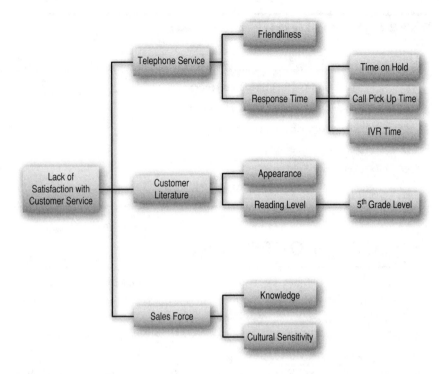

**FIGURE 2-8** CTQ Tree

# COMPLETION OF THE DEFINE PHASE

At the end of the Define Phase, the team should have completed all of the tasks listed in **Table 2-5**. These tasks serve as the basis for the next phase of the project, the Measure Phase.

**Table 2-5** Define Phase checklist

| Done | Task |
|------|------|
| ✔ | Business champion/leader identified |
| ✔ | Team composition complete |
| ✔ | Team members trained on appropriate improvement methods |
| ✔ | Team member participation documented through meeting minutes |

**Table 2-5** Define Phase checklist (*continued*)

| Done | Task |
|------|------|
| ✔ | Project resources identified and secured |
| ✔ | Customers segmented and CTQs identified |
| ✔ | Initial data collection performed |
| ✔ | Project charter completed |
| ✔ | Process map complete |
| ✔ | SIPOC map complete and validated by team and managers |

# DISCUSSION QUESTIONS

1. Describe the project charter. What is the purpose of the project charter? List the major sections of the charter and provide a brief description of each.
2. What is the Voice of the Customer (VOC)? Name three approaches to obtaining the VOC.
3. How is the CAHPS survey used in health care to obtain the VOC? Name three advantages for using the CAHPS survey to understand customers.
4. Name three other methods of listening to customers and provide a brief description of each.
5. What is the Kano Model? How does it help define customer preferences?
6. How does stakeholder analysis support project success? What does a stakeholder matrix show?
7. Describe process mapping. What is the product of process mapping?
8. Create a flowchart of a process that you use in your work.
9. What is the function of the SIPOC process map? How does the map assist project managers with gaining manager buy in?
10. Brainstorming helps teams produce ideas quickly. Describe the brainstorming process and describe variants like brainwriting and nominal group technique. When are these variants appropriate?
11. Multivoting is a list reduction technique used after brainstorming. Describe the multivoting process and how it is applied to prioritization of ideas.

12. Create an affinity diagram after brainstorming for a problem or issue that your organization faces, or select an issue from the following list:
    • How can we improve the way students learn about quality?
    • What can be done about the state of readiness of students for graduation?
    • Why is our staff satisfaction below benchmarks?
    • What things do we need to consider in planning a perfect meeting?
    • What can be done to ensure proper disposal of recyclable material?
    • How can information flow be improved within our organization?
    • What can be done to ensure fast service at the pharmacy prescription counter?
    • What activities should we plan for the company Christmas party?
13. What is Critical to Quality (CTQ)? Describe the methods used to gain CTQ data and how a CTQ tree is created.

## REFERENCES

1. Agency for Healthcare Research and Quality. *CAHPS ambulatory care survey.* Retrieved from https://www.cahps.ahrq.gov/content/products/PROD_AmbCareSurveys.asp.
2. Agency for Healthcare Research and Quality. *CAHPS facility surveys.* Retrieved from https://www.cahps.ahrq.gov/content/products/PROD_FacilitiesSurveys.asp.
3. Agency for Healthcare Research and Quality. *The CAHPS Connection newsletter.* Retrieved from https://www.cahps.ahrq.gov/content/CAHPSConnection/CAHPSConnectionArchives.asp
4. Ramon Magsaysay Award Foundation. (1984). *Biography of Kawakita.* Retrieved from http://www.rmaf.org.ph/Awardees/Biography/BiographyKawakitaJir.htm

# Measure Phase Tools

*"There are two possible outcomes: if the result confirms the hypothesis, then you've made a measurement. If the result is contrary to the hypothesis, then you've made a discovery."*

—Enrico Fermi

*"If you can't describe what you are doing as a process, you don't know what you are doing."*

—W. Edwards Deming

*"Measurement is the first step that leads to control and eventually to improvement. If you can't measure something, you can't understand it. If you can't understand it, you can't control it. If you can't control it, you can't improve it."*

—H. James Harrington

## THE ESSENCE OF THE MEASURE PHASE

Almost inevitably, a project team wants to jump in and get started on improvements as soon as the team-forming process is complete. Indeed, for many quality frameworks, like lean and PDSA, the move from team formation to improvement project design occurs quickly. However, the Six Sigma paradigm requires a few steps prior to implementation of the

**59**

improvement intervention. Because the Six Sigma approach is built on the scientific method, the team must ensure that the project is designed properly to allow statistically significant inferences to be made from the results, which necessitates a good measurement system and valid analyses. The next two phases—Measure and Analyze—ensure the adequacy of the measurement system and analysis for the project that distinguishes Six Sigma from other quality archetypes. Each phase in DMAIC is built on the prior phases, and this orderly sequence of steps ensures a scientifically valid approach to improvement.

Once the process is studied and understood in the Define Phase, the next step in DMAIC is to refine the measurement system and apply it to the current process to determine baseline performance and provide the information used in the next step in DMAIC, the Analyze Phase, which identifies gaps and develops improvement approaches. The goal of the Measure Phase of a Six Sigma DMAIC project is to collect as much information as possible on the target process to understand not just how it works, but also how well it works. Using the process map from the Define Phase, the team gathers baseline data and begins to put it into a format that allows further analysis for identification of opportunities for improvement. Tools used during the Measure Phase include:

- Process maps—PERT chart and deployment flowchart
- Prioritization matrix
- Process cycle efficiency
- Time value analysis
- Pareto charts
- Run charts
- Control charts
- Failure modes and effects criticality analysis (FMECA)

Deliverables from the Measure Phase are used to drive the Analyze Phase:

- Process metrics with operational definitions
- Measurement system analysis
- Data collection and analysis plan
- Baseline performance—often summarized in calculation of process sigma

Six Sigma is based on a fundamental equation:

$$Y = f(x)$$

Where Y is the main outcome variable (e.g., customer satisfaction or some other critical-to-customer (CTC) requirement) and

X represents one or more factors that contribute to that outcome measure (e.g., speed of service, pleasantness of staff, color of product, etc.) The most important of these factors are called **critical X factors**.

The goal of the Measure Phase is to find those critical Xs and determine their relationship to the Y outcome variable. Additionally, the Measure Phase deliverables ensure that each X and the Y outcome metric has an operational definition (i.e., a precise description of the elements of the factor that must be measured, how they are measured, and the tolerance in the measurement system that could lead to errors just from the process of measurement). Most healthcare professionals remember chemistry lab experiments that required highly precise weight measurements that were performed on sophisticated balances that had glass cages to protect against the effects of air movement on the balance. Six Sigma tolerances are very small, and measurement artifacts may create errors; those artifacts must be understood in detail through a process called measurement system analysis. By properly designing the data collection and analysis plan the likelihood of project success being verifiable increases immensely, and the results can then create actionable information for sustained improvement. Finally, using the data collection system, the project team collects and analyzes baseline data for comparison with post-intervention observations that will help indicate success of the project.

# MEASURE PHASE TOOLS

## Process Maps

The process map created during the Define Phase can be further refined during this DMAIC stage. Lean metrics, such as cycle times, can be related to individual process steps, particularly when the quality problem is related to delays and lags in process operations. The team should have begun the task of creating process measures during the Define Phase, and they will be refined using the process map during the Measure Phase. Process experts can help identify key steps on the process maps, and the team should begin looking for process steps that are subject to excessive variation for further analysis. Some of the measures that are developed in this phase will be important to quantifying the variation that becomes the subject of the Analyze and Improve Phases.

### Performance Evaluation and Review Technique (PERT) Chart

Although a standard flowchart is usually sufficient for evaluating improvement opportunities, several other types of flowcharts are available for the analysis. Particularly as the team enters the Measure Phase, process flows that indicate cycle times for each step in the process, along with slack time measurements, can be of value. These diagrams, termed **Program Evaluation and Review Technique (PERT)** charts, provide a way of conveying information for determining cycle times and targeting improvement opportunities. **Figure 3-1** presents two PERT charts created from the flowchart in Figure 2-5. The flowchart shows the process for classifying a patient into one of four tiers for a care management program using two methods: 1) a paper-based Health Risk Assessment survey and 2)

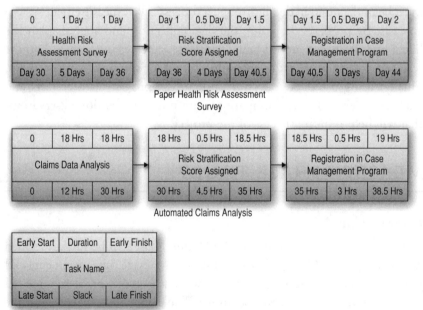

FIGURE 3-1 Program Evaluation and Review Technique chart for diabetic risk stratification

a program using insurance claims data with details of the patient's prior utilization of services. The PERT charts show the shortest path along the top row and the longest path along the bottom row of the cells. The labels for each one of the compartments in the PERT cells are shown in the figure as well. The relationship of the compartments in the cells can be characterized as follows:

- The Earliest Start (ES) of the first cell is usually set at time zero
- The Duration (D) of the step is the best performance time of the step (i.e., the shortest measured time that the step can be completed)
- The Earliest Finish (EF) of the cell is the Earliest Start plus the Duration (EF = ES + D)
- The Latest Start in the first cell is also a measured time and depends on the ability for the process to start on time
- The Slack (S) time represents the time that is wasted in the process and can either be measured by direct observation or by calculation: Slack = Longest Time for the Step − Duration
- The Latest Finish (LF) is the sum of the Latest Start (LS) plus the Duration plus the slack (LF = LS + D + S)
- The Earliest Start of each subsequent cell is the Earliest Finish of the preceding cell
- The Latest Start of each subsequent cell is the Latest Finish of the preceding cell

PERT charts serve nicely as lean management tools, since they readily identify those process steps with prolonged slack times. Some teams use these slack times as leading indicators of potential opportunities for improvement, but a more metric-driven approach digs deeper into process performance using CTQ measures created during the Define Phase and calculating a "sigma level" based on process capability, which we'll discuss later in this chapter.

One particularly important question to resolve in creating the PERT chart is where to obtain the data for the times in the compartments. Most often, these times are collected empirically through direct observation of the process. In Lean terms, this phase would be considered a "walk-around," during which team members observe steps in the process, record times, identify "work-arounds" for bottleneck steps, and find sources of process malfunction. During the walk-around, a checklist should be used to collect time data for each step, consisting of the fastest time and the longest time, from which process duration and slack can be determined. Most of the time, the duration time will be the best time achieved for the step, and the slack time will be derived from the longest time for the step minus the duration. In some cases, however, the best and worst times are "outliers" (i.e., drastically different from typical performance) and in those cases the team may want to use either mean times for duration and slack, or make a cutoff of the times at three standard deviations from the mean as a starting point for the analysis.

### Procedure for PERT Chart

PERT Charts are most easily constructed using software programs that allow manipulation of shapes, such as Microsoft Visio or Microsoft Project. An advantage of Microsoft Project is the ability to change the type of chart relatively simply.

1. Start with a basic flowchart that outlines the steps in the process of interest.
2. Determine the critical path (the sequence of steps required to complete the process) for the process.
3. Use the critical path steps to form the "backbone" of the PERT diagram. Align the steps in the critical path in a straight line using PERT cells as shown in **Figure 3-2**(a).
4. Add times to the critical path nodes as shown in Figure 3-2(b) in accordance with PERT analysis rules.
5. Add subtask nodes to the diagram as they relate to the critical path nodes as indicated in Figure 3-2(c).
6. Add times to each subtask node, ensuring that the subtask times remain consistent with those of the critical path node to which each subtask is related, as in Figure 3-2(d).

The PERT charts in Figures 3-1 and 3-2 were created in Microsoft Visio®, but Microsoft Project® also may be used to construct PERT diagrams (called Network Diagrams in Project). An example PERT chart created in Project can be found in **Figure 3-3**.

(A) Critical Path Steps Arranged in Linear Sequence

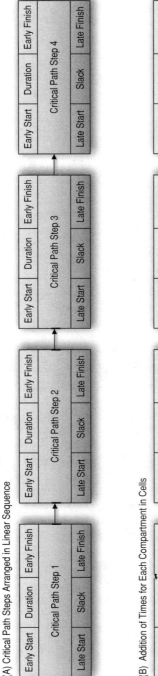

| Early Start | Duration | Early Finish |
|---|---|---|
| | Critical Path Step 1 | |
| Late Start | Slack | Late Finish |

| Early Start | Duration | Early Finish |
|---|---|---|
| | Critical Path Step 2 | |
| Late Start | Slack | Late Finish |

| Early Start | Duration | Early Finish |
|---|---|---|
| | Critical Path Step 3 | |
| Late Start | Slack | Late Finish |

| Early Start | Duration | Early Finish |
|---|---|---|
| | Critical Path Step 4 | |
| Late Start | Slack | Late Finish |

(B) Addition of Times for Each Compartment in Cells

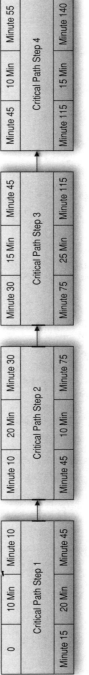
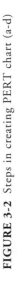
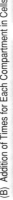

| 0 | 10 Min | Minute 10 |
|---|---|---|
| | Critical Path Step 1 | |
| Minute 15 | 20 Min | Minute 45 |

| Minute 10 | 20 Min | Minute 30 |
|---|---|---|
| | Critical Path Step 2 | |
| Minute 45 | 10 Min | Minute 75 |

| Minute 30 | 15 Min | Minute 45 |
|---|---|---|
| | Critical Path Step 3 | |
| Minute 75 | 25 Min | Minute 115 |

| Minute 45 | 10 Min | Minute 55 |
|---|---|---|
| | Critical Path Step 4 | |
| Minute 115 | 15 Min | Minute 140 |

**FIGURE 3-2** Steps in creating PERT chart (a–d)

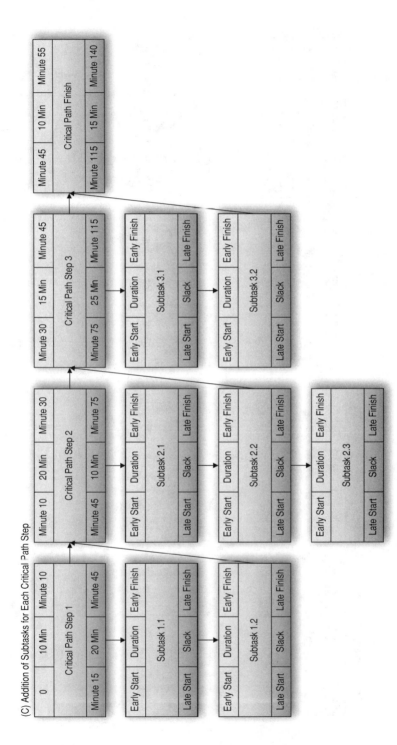

**FIGURE 3-2** Steps in creating PERT chart (a-d) *(continued)*

(D) Add Times for Subtasks, Ensuring That All Times Add Up to The Critical Path and Slack Analysis Totals

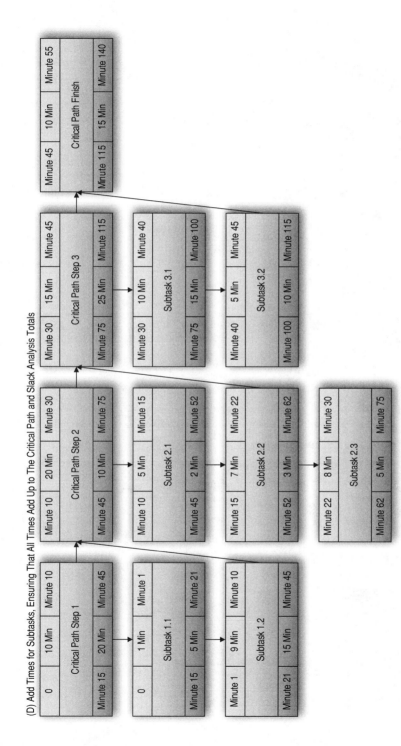

| Minute 15 | 0 | 10 Min | Minute 10 |
|---|---|---|---|
| | Critical Path Step 1 | | |
| Minute 45 | 20 Min | | Minute 45 |

| Minute 15 | 0 | 1 Min | Minute 1 |
|---|---|---|---|
| | Subtask 1.1 | | |
| Minute 21 | 5 Min | | Minute 21 |

| Minute 1 | 9 Min | | Minute 10 |
|---|---|---|---|
| | Subtask 1.2 | | |
| Minute 21 | 15 Min | | Minute 45 |

| Minute 45 | Minute 10 | 20 Min | Minute 30 |
|---|---|---|---|
| | Critical Path Step 2 | | |
| Minute 45 | 10 Min | | Minute 75 |

| Minute 45 | Minute 10 | 5 Min | Minute 15 |
|---|---|---|---|
| | Subtask 2.1 | | |
| Minute 45 | 2 Min | | Minute 52 |

| Minute 15 | 7 Min | | Minute 22 |
|---|---|---|---|
| | Subtask 2.2 | | |
| Minute 52 | 3 Min | | Minute 62 |

| Minute 22 | 8 Min | | Minute 30 |
|---|---|---|---|
| | Subtask 2.3 | | |
| Minute 62 | 5 Min | | Minute 75 |

| Minute 75 | Minute 30 | 15 Min | Minute 45 |
|---|---|---|---|
| | Critical Path Step 3 | | |
| Minute 75 | 25 Min | | Minute 115 |

| Minute 75 | Minute 30 | 10 Min | Minute 40 |
|---|---|---|---|
| | Subtask 3.1 | | |
| Minute 75 | 15 Min | | Minute 100 |

| Minute 100 | Minute 40 | 5 Min | Minute 45 |
|---|---|---|---|
| | Subtask 3.2 | | |
| Minute 100 | 10 Min | | Minute 115 |

| Minute 115 | Minute 45 | 10 Min | Minute 55 |
|---|---|---|---|
| | Critical Path Finish | | |
| Minute 115 | 15 Min | | Minute 140 |

**FIGURE 3-2** Steps in creating PERT chart (a–d) *(continued)*

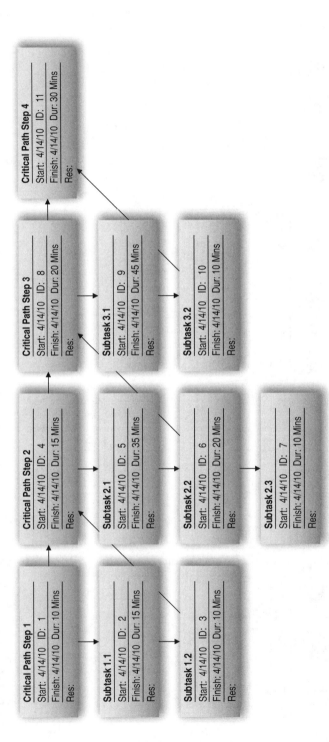

**FIGURE 3-3** PERT(Network) Chart from Microsoft Project™

## Tips and Tricks

- Although the PERT chart cells can have many configurations (note the difference in the cells in Figure 3-2 and 3-3 created in two different software programs), the most useful format is that shown in Figure 3-1, which has all the pertinent times needed to calculate the PERT statistics. Including all the times used in the calculations avoids the need for those using the chart to calculate parameters like the slack time or duration.
- A checklist for calculating PERT statistics can be constructed from an Excel® spreadsheet by listing process steps, and then entering times for each step, including duration and slack times.
- The concept of slack times fits with the lean notion of "nonvalue added" time. Slack times may connote customer wait times, which emanate from a number of sources that are targeted by lean interventions, like transit times, wasted motion, correction and rework, and lack of knowledge at the site of care.

PERT charts have become an important tool for understanding vulnerable steps in a process and selecting targets for improvement. Additionally, the approach provides a concise presentation format for communicating these opportunities to others.

## Deployment Flowchart

Another variation on the basic flowchart is the deployment flowchart, which rearranges the basic flowchart to clarify the individual or department responsible for performing each step in the process. An example of a deployment flowchart can be found in **Figure 3-4**. The deployment flowchart helps each stakeholder and process owner understand responsibilities and accountabilities for process completion. Creation of a deployment flowchart is best performed using a program like Microsoft Visio, which allows rearrangement of shapes as needed for the proper configuration.

These flowcharts not only sequence the activity steps in the process, but they also highlight the interactions between individuals or groups engaged in the process. Each participant's responsibilities are displayed on the process map in a matrix format, clarifying responsibilities and quickly identifying each participant's contribution to the process. This elucidation of accountability has the effect of focusing attention on areas of inefficiency, duplication,

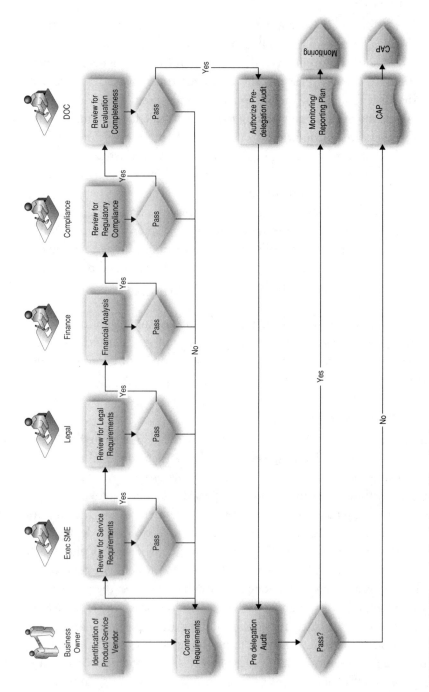

**FIGURE 3-4** PExample Deployment Flowchart

or unnecessary processing (i.e., nonvalue-added work) making them ideal for Lean Six Sigma analyses. Deployment flowcharts are thus useful for determining the staff necessary to perform a process, as well as defining areas of handoffs and transitions that are ready sources of error and waste.

As with other mapping techniques, deployment flowcharts are most useful when they are sufficiently detailed to tell the story of the process. Matching stakeholders with process steps requires accuracy to ensure credibility and to allow correct allocation of resources. Additionally, the flowchart should be as simple as possible to avoid confusion with those who are not deeply familiar with the process. Thus, Albert Einstein's maxim, "Everything should be made as simple as possible, but not simpler," is a good precept to guide creation of the deployment flowchart.

### Procedure for Deployment Flowchart

1. Create an ordered list of process steps, and place a responsible party next to each step. If more than one party is necessary for a step, determine if the parties may be combined into a department or division.
2. Using a program like Microsoft Visio, create a standard flowchart using the steps in the process outlined in step 1.
3. Place the names/positions/department designations in a row across the top of the flowchart.
4. Rearrange the steps in the flowchart into the columns created by the names/positions/departments at the top of the page. As the process steps are moved on the Visio worksheet, the arrows connecting shapes will generally connect automatically in the new flowchart.

### Tips and Tricks

- It is often helpful to color-coded steps related to each stakeholder to simplify interpretation of the chart. For example, Stakeholder 1 may have all related process steps colored blue, Stakeholder 2 may use pink, etc.
- If a process step is performed by more than one stakeholder, and the stakeholders cannot be combined into a functional unit, the step may be replicated in the diagram using the same language for the step, but perhaps customizing the coloring by dividing the box representing the step into a number of sections that may be colored with the shade for each participant. For example, if the process step is performed by

Stakeholders 1 and 2, then half the shape may be colored pink and the other half blue.

- Some deployment flowcharts contain some PERT statistics, like duration of the step and slack time, to provide some guidance regarding the efficiency analysis that may be performed by the team reviewing the flowchart.
- It is often helpful to present the standard flowchart with the deployment flowchart for teams that are not familiar with the latter tool. The standard flowchart helps set the context for the deployment flowchart.
- Transitions and handoffs are key targets for errors, miscommunication, and process failures and are usually the best places to look for opportunities for improvement. The deployment flowchart is an ideal tool for identifying these points.

### Prioritization Matrix

The discussion of brainstorming and multivoting in Chapter 2 described methods of generating ideas and then reducing the large number of ideas into a shortlist of choices based on group consensus. During the Measure Phase, a more quantitative approach to prioritization may be necessary to support decisions for improvement initiatives or establish priorities for measures. The prioritization matrix (PM) is one tool frequently used to achieve more quantifiable rankings for a list of choices. The PM is used for decision support and is sometimes called a decision matrix, and this tool can be used in a number of situations:

- To prioritize complex or unclear issues, where there are multiple criteria for deciding importance
- When there is data available to help score criteria and issues
- To help gain agreement on priorities and key issues for large-scale decisions
- When the extra effort that is required to find a more confident selection than brainstorming alone is considered to be worthwhile

The PM combines a list of elements to be prioritized with weights for each element to create scores for each alternative that can be used to create a ranked list for use in supporting a decision. An example PM is shown in **Figure 3-5** and will be described in more detail in **Scenario 3-1**.

| Average Scores From Survey | | | |
|---|---|---|---|
| | | | |
| Numbers of Patients Impacted | Revenue Potential | Overall Project Cost | Time for Completion |
| 3 | 2 | 2 | 4 |
| 2 | 5 | 3 | 5 |
| 1 | 1 | 4 | 1 |
| 5 | 1 | 1 | 2 |
| 4 | 3 | 3 | 3 |
| 2 | 3 | 5 | 2 |

| Parameter | Numbers of Patients Impacted | Revenue Potential | Overall Project Cost | Time for Completion | |
|---|---|---|---|---|---|
| Weight | 0.15 | 0.4 | 0.3 | 0.15 | |
| | | | | | |
| Unit | Weighted Scores | | | | Total Score |
| ED | 0.45 | 0.8 | 0.6 | 0.6 | 2.45 |
| Obstetrics | 0.3 | 2 | 0.9 | 0.75 | 3.95 |
| Medicine | 0.15 | 0.4 | 1.2 | 0.15 | 1.90 |
| Pediatrics | 0.75 | 0.4 | 0.3 | 0.3 | 1.75 |
| Post-op | 0.6 | 1.2 | 0.9 | 0.45 | 3.15 |
| Neuro | 0.3 | 1.2 | 1.5 | 0.3 | 3.30 |

**FIGURE 3-5** (a) Prioritization Matrix: Raw scores from review team (b) Prioritization Matrix: Weighted scores

## Procedure for Prioritization Matrix

1. Identify the overall objectives for the project (e.g., to determine prioritization for updating inpatient hospital units).
2. Create a task force to work on the issue that includes senior managers, managers from the units or product lines affected, and selected staff.

3. Brainstorm with the task force to identify the parameters to be included and reduce the list to a few critical issues.

4. Create a list of criteria used to judge how well each item on the parameter list serves the project objective. Approaches to identifying criteria may include:
   - Analyze objectives (e.g., optimizing patient satisfaction, reducing operational costs, lower medical safety risk, etc.)
   - Identify practical constraints (e.g., timeline for completion, cost of change, skilled staff availability)
   - Measurability of criterion—can the item be measured objectively or must it be subjectively evaluated.

5. Allocate a weight number to each criterion based on relative importance in achieving the overall objective. Weights may be any range of numbers as long as the relative importance is maintained. For example, in Figure 3-5 the weight for number of patients impacted (0.15) is half that of overall project cost (0.30). The numbers could just as easily have been 15 and 30, rather than the decimals. Weights may be established by the group or by senior managers, or in some cases, by customers through surveys.

6. Determine how the parameters to be used for the decision will be evaluated and scored. Approaches may include:
   - Use a Likert scale (1–5 or 1–10) to indicate how closely the parameter meets the criteria for each alternative in the list; each team member or an expert panel may review the alternatives and parameters and score each item using the scale.
   - Use a voting system in which each reviewer has a fixed number of points to distribute across items. For example, each reviewer may have 100 points that are distributed among all the alternatives and parameters.
   - Use negative scores for negative effects, changing the Likert scale to a range of −5 to +5. For example, if the cost of the project for one alternative exceeds budget, it may receive a −3 score.

7. Choose a review team to score each parameter for each alternative. The team may be constituted from the project team, managers, or an outside group with particular expertise.

8. Enter each score into the raw score matrix (Figure 3-5[a]), and then multiply each score by the weight allocated to the parameter to get

the weighted score for each parameter for each alternative as in Figure 3-5(b). Spreadsheet programs make this process very easy.

9. Add the weighted scores for each alternative (row) and total as in Figure 3-5(b). The Total Score column in Figure 3-5(b) represents the sum of each row and the final prioritization scores for the alternatives.

10. The final list of prioritized items may be made clearer for communication and decision making by sorting it into priority order and displaying it in a Pareto chart as shown in **Figure 3-6** and discussed later in this chapter.

### Tips and Tricks

- Weighting in the prioritization matrix may seem like a daunting task, but often the weights are set by senior managers at the outset of the project, as the project plan is being developed during the Define Phase. If senior managers have delegated the task to the project team, then other sources of weighting include the process owners, customers, and subject matter experts. In most cases, a short survey can collect

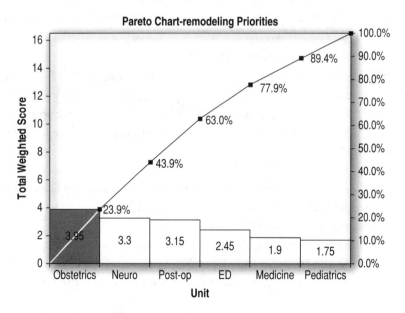

**FIGURE 3-6** Pareto Chart for Remodeling Project

the data necessary to establish weights. For example, a four question survey that collects data on the importance of each of the parameters on a five-point Likert scale can usually settle the issue, and in some cases, adding an additional set of questions regarding the organization's performance to the survey provides the information needed to calculate a score that reflects both the importance of an item, as well as how well the organization currently performs that function.

## Process Cycle Efficiency (Value Added Ratio)

This metric allows managers to understand process efficiency from the standpoint of value added work. As teams begin to formulate strategies for improvement during the Measure Phase, multiple metrics will be considered. One of the most useful high-level measures is process cycle efficiency, defined as follows:

$$\text{PCE} = \frac{\text{Value added work}}{\text{Total work}} = 1 - \frac{\text{Nonvalue added work}}{\text{Total work}}$$

The variables in the equation can be defined in several different ways (e.g., as times, labor and material costs, or other inputs relating to work performed) but the PCE is a decimal that is usually converted to a percentage.

### Procedure for Process Cycle Efficiency

The PCE calculation requires a flowchart (preferably a PERT chart or value stream map, or VSM) as a starting point. Although the VSM is the preferred tool of Lean practitioners, a PERT chart is an effective approach, as well. Once the PERT chart has been developed, the procedure for determining PCE involves:

1. Add up the total time required for the process, called the Lead Time, or sometimes the Production Lead Time (PLT).
2. Add up the total nonvalue added time.
3. Divide the nonvalue added time by the total process time.
4. Subtract the resulting ratio from 1.
5. Convert the resulting fraction to a percentage by multiplying by 100.

For example, consider the generic PERT chart in **Figure 3-7**. Recall that the row of times across the top represents the most efficient process time,

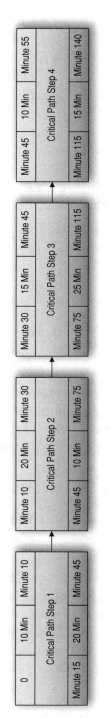

**FIGURE 3-7** Generic PERT chart for PCE

while the row of times across the bottom denotes the least efficient process time (i.e., the process time with slack times added in). The slack time is the value in the center cell of the bottom row. Thus, to calculate the PCE, the slack times are summed:

$$20 \text{ min} + 10 \text{ min} + 25 \text{ min} + 15 \text{ min} = 70 \text{ min}$$

That sum is then divided by the total process time for the bottom row (i.e., the least efficient process time):

$$\frac{70 \text{ min}}{155 \text{ min}} = 0.45$$

This ratio represents the proportion of nonvalue added time, and to calculate the value added ratio, it must be subtracted from 1, as follows:

$$1 - 0.45 = .55$$

Finally, the proportion is converted to a percentage by multiplying by 100:

$$PCE = 100 \times 0.55 = 55\%$$

Thus, the process in Figure 3-7 has only 55% of its time in actually producing value, and 45% of the time nonvalue added work is being performed. This ratio can be used to approximate the cost of the nonvalue added time, as well. Assume that analysis of the process has determined the following:

- Labor costs per cycle = $4,500
- Materials costs per cycle = $3,500
- Allocated overhead costs per cycle = $2,000
- Total costs per cycle = $10,000

Since nonvalue added work consumes 45% of the overall work, the team can estimate that about $4,500 is being wasted with each cycle of the process. It is important to remember that this number is only an estimate, since the actual work lost varies in each step, and the cost of each step is not uniform.

## Tips and tricks for PCE

1. The PCE is a high level metric for overall process efficiency. As Figure 3-7 shows, the efficiency of each step varies considerably, and so the "drill down" for a low PCE is the evaluation of each step to determine the locus for nonvalue added time.

2. PCE values for each of an organization's processes prove useful for management scorecards. Since they are high level measures, they can help managers hone in on less effective processes to allocate scarce improvement resources. The next level in the analysis, however, entails understanding the costs of improving each process along with the expected incremental increase in PCE and other metrics.

# TIME VALUE ANALYSIS (TVA)

This lean tool helps teams understand the relative influence of Value Added (VA) and Nonvalue Added (NVA) time for each step in a process using a graphic display of the two measures. The stacked bar graph for the TVA provides rapid insight into the steps in the process that have more NVA than VA, thus more effectively identifying targets for intervention.

### Procedure for Time Value Analysis

Calculation of the parameters needed to create a TVA chart is relatively straightforward. Using the PERT chart in **Figure 3-7** again, the NVA time equates to the slack time, and the VA time is the process time in the middle cell of the top row (labeled "duration" in the PERT definitions). These numbers are then used as follows:

1. A table of values is entered into Excel using the duration (value added) and slack (nonvalue added) times

2. The table is used to create a stacked bar graph, like that shown in **Figure 3-8** that used data from Figure 3-7.

The TVA graph is useful for teams that are working to identify targets for intervention, as well as reporting to senior managers.

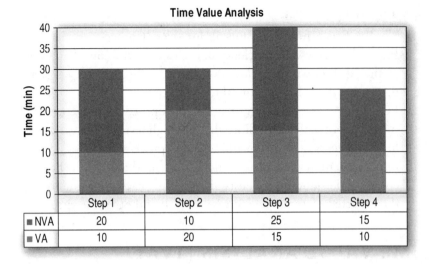

| | Step 1 | Step 2 | Step 3 | Step 4 |
|---|---|---|---|---|
| ■ NVA | 20 | 10 | 25 | 15 |
| ■ VA | 10 | 20 | 15 | 10 |

**FIGURE 3-8**  Time Value Analysis

## Tips and tricks

1. TVA charts provide two important pieces of information—the division of VA and NVA times for each step, and the total time that each step contributes to the process. The more complex steps often consume the greatest time, but that is not always the case. Sometimes a step with a large amount of NVA is apparent on the NVA, such as Step 3 in Figure 3-7. That situation almost always connotes "low hanging fruit" and an opportunity to make substantial improvements with little investment in time and money.

2. Another situation that often warrants intervention is that in Step 1, where the NVA is almost twice the VA. In that circumstance, targeting the NVA with lean analyses and interventions can allow the team to make substantial gains without a lot of resources.

## Pareto Charts

Almost everyone is familiar with the Pareto principle—80% of effects come from 20% of causes. This widely used principle, often called the

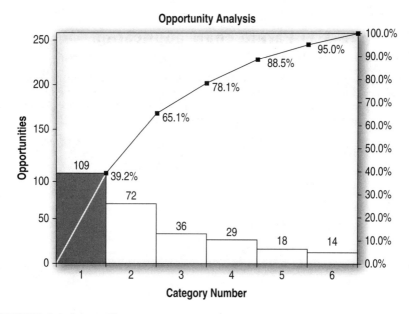

**FIGURE 3-9** Pareto Chart

80–20 rule, helps to quickly visualize the most important elements of a process that present the best targets for improvement initiatives. A representative Pareto chart is shown in **Figure 3-9**. The vertical axis on the left side of the graph measures the frequency of occurrence, which is the count of the number of times that an event or measure occurs, and this parameter is represented by the bars on the graph. The bars can also represent cost or any other numeric metric. The linear plot on the graph is measured on the right vertical axis and is the cumulative percentage of the total number of occurrences. The traditional Pareto chart places the occurrences in decreasing order to produce the familiar pattern seen in Figure 3-9. Thus, the graph in the figure demonstrates that the first three categories of opportunities involve 78% of the potential options and will likely yield the greatest return on investment for improvement initiatives.

# Example 3-1: Pareto chart application to medication errors

Carl Curative, the pharmacy director at AAA Clinics, has tracked pharmacy errors in his facility for the past several months and is trying to determine the best way to spend his limited funds on eliminating these errors. He classified the errors into five categories and created the following table of drug event frequencies:

| Issue | Number |
|---|---|
| Handwriting | 68 |
| Decimal point | 12 |
| Weight dose | 70 |
| Bedside administration | 5 |
| Dose timing | 52 |
| Wrong patient | 5 |
| Wrong medication | 22 |
| Drug-drug interaction | 35 |
| Avoidable side effect | 23 |

Using the Pareto chart function in QI Macros (a Microsoft Excel® add-in), Carl created a Pareto chart of medication events as shown in **Figure 3-10**.

The Pareto chart provides a convenient display of the drug events with frequencies and percentages that indicate the top 77% of causes include four categories: dose calculations based on weight, handwriting, dose timing (too early or too late), and drug-drug interactions. Carl convened an improvement team to begin focusing on these four top issues.

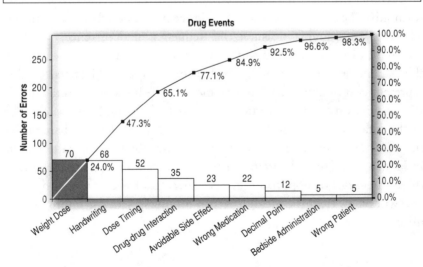

**FIGURE 3-10** Pareto Chart of Drug Events

Pareto charts help focus improvement efforts on the most important issues among a potentially large number of factors. In situations like Example 3-1, the Pareto chart can help a team avoid wasted time and resources as it attempts to direct attention to the most critical elements of a process that will generate the greatest improvements. Numerous programs can generate these charts, making them one of the most straightforward methods that a team can use to prioritize project issues.

### Tips and Tricks

1. Although these charts can be created on an Excel® bar chart template, most users find it easier to use statistical software or Excel® add-ins like QI Macros.
2. As the team begins to consider collecting data to determine project priorities, careful consideration should be given to the categories for the data. As often as possible, categories should be selected that are standard in the industry. For example, the categories for the medication events in Example 3-1 are commonly used types of errors in drug evaluation reviews. Using standardized categories will allow benchmarking in many cases and allow the team to set realistic targets for improvement.

## Run Charts

Many measures are tracked over time using simple graphs that plot the measure on the y-axis and time on the x-axis. Statisticians have created a number of rules for these trend charts, based on the characteristics of sequences of points. The resulting chart, which plots the data points on a chart with the median of all the points, is called a run chart. A sample run chart is shown in **Figure 3-11**.

### Procedure for Run Chart

1. Data points are plotted for each time period on a line chart.
2. A line representing the median is added to the graph to facilitate runs analysis.
3. Runs are identified as one or more consecutive points on either side of the center line. Points on the median are not counted. In most cases, runs are circled on the chart, as shown in **Figure 3-12**. The pattern of runs on the chart indicates the presence of special cause variation or common cause variation.

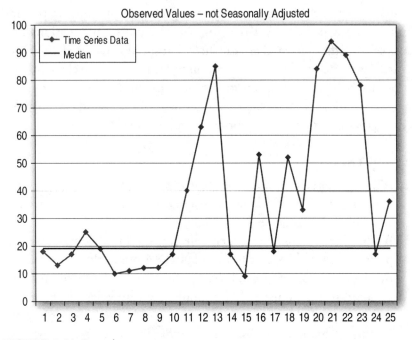

**FIGURE 3-11** Run chart

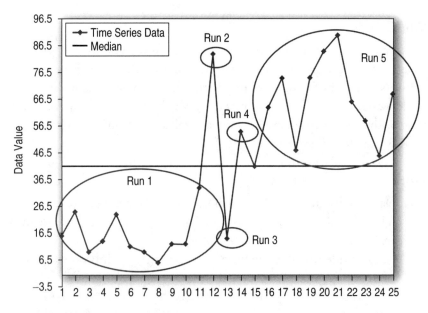

**FIGURE 3-12** Run chart with runs identified

4. Once the runs are identified, statistical tests can be applied to determine if they fall into common or special cause variation categories. With 25 data points, statistical patterns can be discerned that might indicate whether a data value is due to inherent variation in the process (common cause) or some new or external factor (special cause).

Special cause variation arises from an unusual circumstance, such as an automobile crash bringing a surge of patients to the emergency department or an influenza pandemic increasing the hospital census. Special causes create process instability and therefore unpredictable results; thus, actions that may be undertaken to improve the process may not produce predictable results, but may instead only increase variation and waste. Special cause variation is best managed by applying the root cause analysis (RCA) approach, defining the underlying cause(s) of the aberrant result, and then targeting interventions to resolve the unusual cause.

Common cause variation, on the other hand, indicates that the process is designed to allow a level of variation that may add to cost and not quality. As will be seen in the discussion on control charts, common cause variation indicates that data points fall within $\pm3$ sigma limits of the process mean. In this situation, managers must determine if the variation is sufficient to warrant process redesign interventions that consume time and cost money or if the process simply needs to be monitored to assure that it remains in control. The costs of any interventions must be offset by cost savings in the process or production of a higher quality service/product that can command a higher price.

Special cause variation is detected on a run chart by performing a three step "runs analysis" using the following three tests:

1. **Evaluation of variability**—in this test, the number of runs is counted to determine if there are either too many or too few runs. Based on the number of points in the run chart, a statistical prediction can be made of the total number of runs expected (**Table 3-1**). **Figure 3-12** shows five runs, while the table indicates that for 25 points, at least nine runs would be expected; thus, the first runs test indicates a special cause is present in the process.
2. **Evaluation of process shift**—indicated by too many points in a run, the process shift shows that the underlying process has changed or that there is a special cause present. For runs of 20 or more points,

**Table 3-1** Run chart probability table

| Number of points excluding points on the median | Lower limit for number of runs | Upper limit for number of runs |
|:---:|:---:|:---:|
| 14 | 4 | 11 |
| 15 | 4 | 12 |
| 16 | 5 | 12 |
| 17 | 5 | 13 |
| 18 | 6 | 13 |
| 19 | 6 | 14 |
| 20 | 6 | 15 |
| 21 | 7 | 15 |
| 22 | 7 | 16 |
| 23 | 8 | 16 |
| 24 | 8 | 17 |
| 25 | 9 | 17 |
| 26 | 9 | 18 |
| 27 | 9 | 19 |
| 28 | 10 | 19 |
| 29 | 10 | 20 |
| 30 | 11 | 21 |

Based on: Swed, F. & Eisenhart, C. (1943). Tables for testing randomness of groupings in a sequence of alternatives. *Annals of Mathematical Statistics*, 14, 66–87.
Values found in: Joint Commission Resources, Inc. (2001). *Managing performance measurement data in health care*, (p. 66). Chicago, IL: Joint Commission Resources Publications.

a run of eight points can indicate a process shift, and for runs of less than 20 points, the generally accepted test is seven points in a run. In Figure 3-12, Run 1 has 11 points and Run 5 has 12 points, indicating special cause variation.

3. **Evaluation of trend**—most quality professionals consider at least seven or eight consecutive points upward or downward as an indication of a trend on a run chart. For the trend analysis, points on the median count as well. In Figure 3-12, starting with Run 3 and continuing through Run 5, the data indicates a clear upward trend of 13 points.

## Tips and tricks

1. Run charts, like Pareto charts, can be created in Excel without special software, but most statistical process control (SPC) software programs not only create the run chart, but also apply the runs analysis to the chart. Thus, for most practitioners, an SPC software package makes the task easier and less prone to error.

2. Although many different runs analysis tests may be used to analyze run charts, the three tests noted here are the easiest to apply and are very reliable in picking up special cause variation. More detailed analysis can be performed using control charts, as described in the next section.

3. Control charts generally require 20 points to ensure statistical validity, and so run charts are often used in the early phase of process analysis when fewer than 20 data points are available.

4. In some cases, the run chart trend suggests a relationship between the measurement variable and the time variable. In those cases, addition of a trend line, such as that in **Figure 3-13**, can help better understand the relationship using linear regression analysis. Strong correlations may suggest that the process is indeed changing over

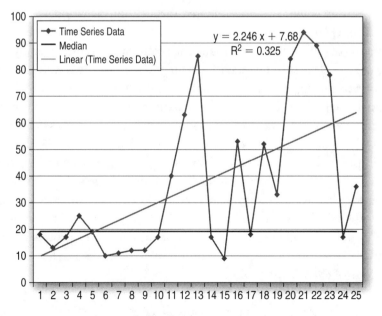

**FIGURE 3-13** Run chart with trendline

time and may prompt further evaluation of the process to determine if the change is intended.

## Control Charts

Control charts were developed by a physicist and statistician, Dr. Walter Shewhart, while he worked at Bell Labs in the 1920s. Bell Telephone was trying to reduce the frequency of costly maintenance for buried telephone cables by improving the reliability of the cable manufacturing process. Shewhart introduced the concepts of common cause and special cause variation, as well as the use of control charts to graphically evaluate performance and variation. With that relatively simple concept, the science of statistical process control was born. The most important consequence of the concept for Bell Labs was the ability to improve prediction of future output and costs by bringing a production process into statistical control (i.e., demonstrating only common cause variation in the process). Additionally, Dr. Shewhart used statistical theory to demonstrate that data from physical processes follow a normal distribution, validating the statistical significance of control charts for scientifically predicting process performance. Before long, other quality engineers, like W. Edwards Deming, discovered the value of statistical process control, and the science of quality improvement was disseminated throughout the world.

Control charts are special versions of run charts, and they provide additional ways of differentiating common cause from special cause variation. The value of control charts is to establish if a process is in control (i.e., if all points fall between the upper and lower control limits). In that event, the variation from point to point is considered common cause and due to "normal" process variation. Special cause variation is connoted by any observations outside the control limits or systematic patterns (runs) inside control limits, and this variance is usually due to a new, unanticipated aberration. Since increased variation means increased cost of poor quality (COPQ), a special cause point on the control chart requires immediate investigation using techniques like Root Cause Analysis (RCA). As such, it adds a level of discipline to the improvement process that allows more aggressive management of process quality. **Figure 3-14** provides a sample of a control chart known as a c-chart.

A control chart consists of:

- Data points representing a measure of a quality characteristic in samples taken from the process at different times

- The mean of the metric calculated from all the samples used for the chart drawn as the center line, or CL
- Upper and lower control limits that indicate the limits for "common cause" variation, usually drawn at ±3 sigma, or three standard deviations from the mean

The chart In Figure 3-14 has a number of other lines, as well. These extra lines are drawn at ±1 sigma and ±2 sigma levels which divide the common cause area into zones, as noted on the chart. Rules have been created that help with interpretation of special causes. By default, Zone A is defined as the area between 2 and 3 sigma on both sides of the center line; Zone B is defined as the area between 1 and 2 sigma; and Zone C is defined as the area between the center line and 1 sigma. Rules regarding runs of points in these zones provide early notification of special cause process variability and can signal a need to increase the rate of sample measurement to determine if the process is deteriorating.

It should be clear by now that control limits are very important decision aids, since they define the limits of expected process behavior. Importantly, though, upper and lower control limits have no inherent relationship to specifications like regulatory requirements or accreditation standards. In many cases, the process mean (i.e., the center line) may not even be the same as the target value of the quality measure; in these

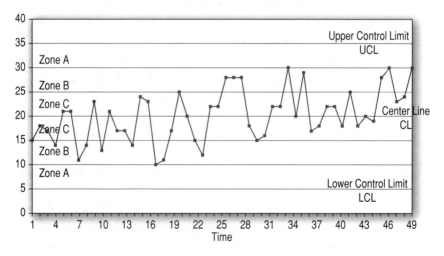

**FIGURE 3-14** Example C-chart control chart

situations, the process design may be fundamentally incapable of meeting customer requirements, which may necessitate drastic changes to improve performance to the point of delivering services or products that are acceptable. The alternative (i.e., trying to make an existing process perform at a level for which it is not designed) usually leads to greater variation, lower efficiency, and higher costs. Thus, the best alternative to a process that is performing at a level that does not meet specifications is to redesign the process so that the expected performance (the measurement data centers on the mean performance of the process) meets the customer's requirements.

Sigma levels represent an estimate of the standard deviation based on the type of data being collected and analyzed. Thus, the 3 sigma control limits on either side of the mean create boundaries for common cause variation that contain 99.7% of the data points from a process. The chance that a process data point would fall outside the 3 sigma control limits is thus only 3 chances in 1000 which is sufficient to reduce the likelihood of "tampering," or treating a common cause data point like a special cause and taking the wrong approach to trying to improve the process. Control charts are constructed using rigorous statistical rules, but many statistical software programs like SAS, SPSS, and Minitab, as well as statistical add-ins for Excel like QI Macros, create these charts quite nicely.

### Control Chart Selection

Although control charts have a fairly standard format, there are a number of different types because of the differences in statistical approaches to create the control limits. The selection diagram for different types of control charts can be found in **Figure 3-15**.

The selection process starts with the type of data in the measurement set. From a statistical perspective, there are two types of data that can be analyzed:

- Attributes data—data that is represented in discrete units (dollars, hours, deaths, number of patients seen, number of no-shows, yes-no options) which measure the presence or absence of an attribute or characteristic; attributes data consists of integers or sometimes ratios of integers.
- Continuous data—usually associated with some sort of physical measurement, continuous data can conceptually take on any value inside some interval; continuous data is considered to be a value in the set of real numbers.

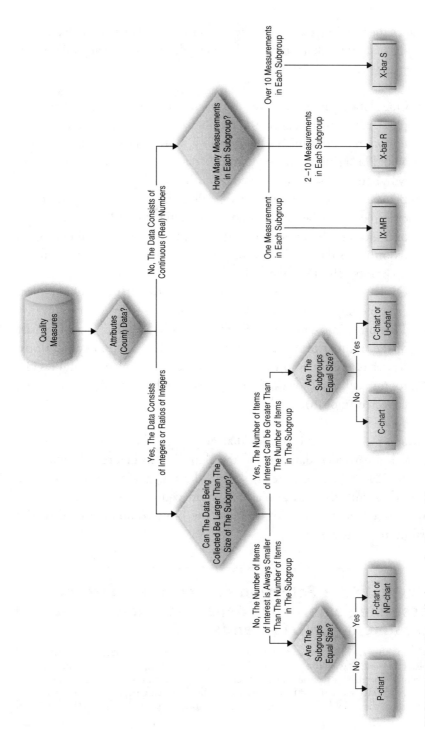

**FIGURE 3-15** Control chart selection decision tree

Once the type of data is clear, the decision tree can be used to determine the type of control chart to be used. Data collections generally follow just a few patterns:

- One data point is collected for each time period. For example, a physicians' office collects the number of patients who do not show up for an appointment each day for a month (no-shows). That data would be a single integer (attributes data) for each time period (day) with about 30 points collected (month).
- Between 2 and 9 data points are collected for each time period. An example might be daily blood sugar values for a diabetic collected over a 6-month period. The data would be 7 values of blood sugars (continuous data) collected for each time period (week) with about 26 points collected (6 months).
- Over 9 data points are collected for each time period. One typical example might be the number of cleaning issues in each room in a 12-room clinic collected daily for a month. The data would consist of the number of defects (cleaning issues like unclean countertops, wastebaskets not emptied, etc.) for a specific number of samples (12 rooms) collected for each time period (daily) with about 30 points collected (month).

Many programs have wizards that help select the appropriate control chart for a particular data set, but the algorithm in Figure 3-15 will provide guidance when software does not make a suggestion. Although other types of control charts are available for more complex situations, the seven charts noted on the decision tree are the most commonly used in the healthcare industry.

---

## Example 3-2 Selection of a control chart for assessing emergency department left without treatment (LWOT) trends

The ED supervisor at University Hospital wanted to determine patterns in patient visits that ended with the patient being triaged, but leaving before treatment had been rendered. These patients were often tired of waiting and decided to leave before they were evaluated by the physician, but after being triaged by the nurse, and since they could not be billed they represented a significant loss of revenue.

The supervisor felt that if she could determine patterns of LWOT patients and avoid overestimating the number by reviewing special causes, she would be able to schedule nursing staff more effectively and reduce the number of LWOT patients. She used the ED patient visit log, and analyzed data for a month. She was familiar with the effect that special causes can change the number of ED visits and LWOT patients quickly. For example, last month, a 10-car pileup on the interstate highway brought 35 casualties to the department for treatment. Since the supervisor wanted to staff the department as lean as possible, she decided to use a control chart to quickly identify those special causes and avoid overestimates of staffing needs. She will use the ratio of LWOT to COMPLETED visits for the control chart.

To determine which type of control chart to use, she turned to the decision tree in Figure 3-15. The first decision regards the type of data, which in this case is the count of visits per day and the number of LWOT patients per day, which connotes attributes data. Since this data set will be a daily ratio of two counts, each data point will consist of a single day, so all of the subgroups (single days) are of equal size. Since the LWOT patients could potentially exceed the number of completed visits, the selection arm for C- and U-charts is selected. Finally, since subgroups (i.e., number of visits each day) can vary, the best chart for this application is the C-chart.

## Interpretation of the Control Chart

Control charts provide two types of information for the quality team: performance of the mean relative to a specification value and the amount of variation in the process. Nearly every process has a required level of performance that can be measured. The measurements become data points on the control chart, and the average (or mean) of the data points is the center line (CL) of the control chart. The difference between the process mean (CL) and the required level of performance provides basic information on process capability. If the difference is substantial, then variation is also typically very high as process owners try to meet process variation through disjointed approaches to process improvement.

So the next step in control chart review is an assessment of variation. There are at least three different sets of rules for interpreting variation and identifying special causes, but the most commonly used is the Western Electric rule set outlined in **Table 3-2**.

A point or run that satisfies any of the four rules can be designated a special cause and investigated as such using tools like Root Cause Analysis. There is always a possibility of a false positive (i.e., an indication of a special cause when one does not exist). The chances of a false positive assessment are relatively small, but not zero. False positive estimates for the Western Electric rules are about one in 91.75 observations when all four

**Table 3-2** Western Electric rules for control chart interpretation

| Rule | Definition |
|---|---|
| 1 | Any single data point falls outside the 3σ limit from the center line (i.e., any point that falls outside Zone A, beyond either the upper or lower control limit) |
| 2 | Two out of three consecutive points fall beyond the 2σ limit (in Zone A or beyond), on the same side of the centerline |
| 3 | Four out of five consecutive points fall beyond the 1σ limit (in Zone B or beyond), on the same side of the center line |
| 4 | Nine consecutive points fall on the same side of the center line (in Zone C or beyond) |

Data from: Western Electric Company, Statistical Quality Control Handbook, 1984, AT&T, Indianapolis, IN.

rules are applied to the control chart. One way to reduce the chance of false positives (Type I errors in statistical terms) is to ensure that the rules for evaluating the chart are selected before the data are plotted.

### Tips and tricks

1. In some cases, a special cause may not be of sufficient magnitude for the chart to produce an immediate out of control condition. If there is reason to believe that a special cause is occurring, the team may want to collect more data for a short period of time or use another type of control chart, such as a CUSUM or exponentially weighted moving average chart that detects out of control points earlier.

2. When a special cause is detected, the logical approach to determining the issue(s) contributing to the out of control point is a RCA. Unfortunately, the team often focuses on one issue and misses a number of other problems that also contributed to the event. For example, the ED may attribute an out of control spike in the LWOT rate one day because of a train wreck, but in fact a number of operational issues, such as traffic patterns in the ED, supply availability, staffing patterns, and equipment may also be related. Investigation of a special cause should avoid narrow reviews and include all possible underlying issues.

3. Sometimes the Individual X-Moving Range (IX-MR) chart can be used for attributes data. For example, when the quality metric is counting the number of nonconformities, which usually connotes the use of the np-chart for attributes data, an alternative method of analyzing and graphing the points on a control chart would be to use

the IX-MR chart. Although this approach violates the decision tree, it is acceptable from a statistical standpoint and often easier for staff to understand if the most common charts used are for continuous data.

## Failure Mode and Effects Criticality Analysis (FMECA)

The FMECA is also used to prioritize potential causes of failure so that a team may develop and implement preventive actions, and the approach prioritizes process risks by calculation of a criticality score. FMECA (also sometimes shortened to FMEA) is a stepwise approach to pinpoint all possible failures in a design or in an existing process, and the approach has been used in manufacturing and service industries to improve the safety of a product or service. It has become a relative mainstay in health care since The Joint Commission began requiring it as part of its quality standards several years ago.

"Failure modes" connote the ways, or modes, by which a step in the process or a resulting product or service might fail. Failures include any potential or actual errors or defects, particularly those that affect the customer. "Effects analysis" refers to collecting data and assessing the consequences of failures. During FMECA, failures are prioritized by three important parameters:

- Seriousness of the consequences
- Frequency of failures
- Ease of detection of each failure

Once process failures are prioritized, the next steps in FMECA involve developing process improvements to eliminate or reduce each failure in order of priority. The Criticality Scores calculated as part of the FMECA process help to verify current improvement efforts to better understand which interventions have produced changes that enhance the product or service. Later in the continuous improvement cycle, FMECA can be used for process control, making the approach a useful tool throughout the life cycle of a product or service.

### When to Use FMECA

FMECA is a tool that is best applied in specific circumstances:

- For process, product, or service design or redesign
- For new applications of an existing process, product or service

- Prior to developing control plans for a new or modified process
- Planning improvement goals for an existing process, product, or service
- To analyze failures in an existing process, product, or service
- As a preventive measure during the life cycle of a process, product, or service

These applications of the technique demonstrate the utility of the FMECA approach. In health care, FMECA is most frequently used to examine existing processes to identify potential patient safety issues.

### FMECA Procedure

The process for FMECA is well characterized and consists of the steps in **Table 3-3**. Calculation of the criticality score from the FMECA is detailed in **Table 3-4**.

Note that the FMECA process is designed to follow the form in Table 3-4, and so the process can be documented fully by using that form.

The criticality analysis, which involves calculation of the Risk Priority Number (RPN) is relatively straightforward, but it is also a powerful way to assign priorities in the Measure and Analyze Phases of DMAIC. Since the RPN is a multiplied value, the higher the RPN, the greater the risk of failure that causes substantial customer harm. Thus, the RPN values can be used by improvement teams to prioritize issues for improvement interventions as shown in Example 3-3.

---

## Example 3-3 Using the RPN

The 4-West (orthopedics) nursing performance improvement team has committed to improving their Falls With Injury rates, and so they outlined the entire process of daily patient care for their highest risk patients, those with hip fracture repairs. They brainstormed failure modes for each step in the process, assigned Severity, Occurrence, and Detection scores that were used to calculate RPN values for each step in the care process, resulting in the data in **Table 3-5**.

The RPN values were calculated according to the standard formula, and as is quite evident, two steps in the process (steps numbered 7 and 10) stand out in terms of priorities for intervention. The team then concentrated their efforts on the afternoon free time and the overnight time period.

**Table 3-3** FMECA procedure

| Step | Description | Comment |
|---|---|---|
| 1. | Assemble team | • Cross-functional team with knowledge about the process, product, or service and customer needs<br>• Roles may include nurses, environmental staff, administration, billing, finance, technicians, physicians, therapists, and materials managers |
| 2. | Identify scope | • Boundaries for project<br>• Level of detail required for analysis<br>• Flowcharts can characterize the process and help set the scope<br>• Ensure that all team members understand the scope |
| 3. | Complete FMECA form | • Using the form in Table 3-4, complete the identifying information for the FMECA project in the header portion |
| 4. | Determine functions related to scope | • Purpose of target system or process<br>• Voice of the Customer<br>• Break the system or process into subunits for analysis of functions |
| 5. | Identify all possible failure modes | • Brainstorm potential failures with experienced team members<br>• Record all potential failure modes in the template |
| 6. | Identify consequences of each failure mode | • Determine all downstream effects of failure mode on other systems and the customer, including regulatory issues, legal and ethical problems<br>• Determine effect on customers of the failure mode |
| 7. | Determine severity score | • Use the rating scale in the template for the severity rating (S)<br>• Severity rating scale ranges from 1 to 10, where 1 is lowest significance and 10 is catastrophic<br>• Use the highest S for failure modes that have more than one effect |
| 8. | Determine root causes | • Perform RCA for each failure mode to determine all potential root causes<br>• List all possible causes for each failure mode on the FMECA form |

**Table 3-3**  FMECA procedure (*continued*)

| Step | Description | Comment |
|---|---|---|
| 9. | Determine occurrence score | • For each failure mode cause, determine the occurrence rating (O), which is an estimate of the probability of failure occurring for the listed reason<br>• Use the occurrence rating scale on the template with a range from 1 to 10, where 1 is extremely unlikely and 10 is virtually certain<br>• Enter the O in the appropriate column on the template |
| 10. | Identify current process interventions | • For each failure mode cause, identify current process interventions that are currently in place to keep failures from reaching customers<br>• The interventions may include detection of failures that reached the customer, as well as preventive measures |
| 11. | Determine detection rating (D) | • For each failure mode, estimate the detection rating (D) to assess the ability of the process or system to detect the failure mode after it has happened before the customer is affected.<br>• Use the scale on the template for D, which is ranked from 1 (detection is certain) to 10 (detection is certain not to occur) |
| 12. | Assign a critical Characteristic | • Using the ratings on the template, assign a critical characteristic, which is an indicator that reflects safety or compliance with regulatory or accreditation requirements<br>• If a critical characteristic is assigned, then S is usually 9–10, O is above 3, and D is above 3 |
| 13. | Calculate the Risk Priority Number (RPN) and Criticality | • RPN = S × O × D<br>• Criticality = S × O<br>• RPN and criticality help prioritize potential failures |
| 14. | Identify recommended actions | • Actions are design or process changes to lower severity or occurrence, or improve detection before a problem reaches a customer<br>• Assign responsibility for the actions and target completion dates |
| 15. | Track action completion and recalculate RPN | • As actions are completed, document results and completion dates<br>• Reassign S, O, and D ratings and recalculate RPNs |

## Table 3-4  FMECA data template

| Failure mode and effects criticality analysis | | | | | | |
|---|---|---|---|---|---|---|
| FMECA start date: | | FMECA end date: | | | Page number | |
| Target process | | Team leader: | | | | |
| Team members: | | Process owner: | | | | |

| Process Step | Quality/safety requirements | Failure mode | Failure effects | Severity score | Class of severity | Causes / mechanisms of failure |
|---|---|---|---|---|---|---|
| <Step number on the flowchart> | <Definition of quality or safety requirements described in detail> | <Methods by which the process step could fail; issues that could cause failure> | <Downstream effects of the failure, including effects on customers; level of effect (i.e., the severity of the effect on specific constituencies)> | 1 = No effect<br>2 = Very minor<br>3 = Minor<br>4 = Very low<br>5 = Low loss<br>6 = Moderate loss<br>7 = High loss<br>8 = Very high loss<br>9 = Hazardous with warning<br>10 = Hazardous without warning | Critical<br>Key<br>Major<br>Significant | <Listing of all potential causes of each failure mode> |

| | | | | | | | | | Post-action follow up | | | | | |
|---|---|---|---|---|---|---|---|---|---|---|---|---|---|---|
| Occurrence score | Current interventions | Current measures to detect failure mode | Detection score | Risk priority number (RPN) | Recommended action(s) | Responsibility for completion | Target completion date | Actions taken | Date complete | Severity | Occurrence | Detection | RPN |
| 1 = Very low (<1/10,000,000)<br>2 = Low (1/1,000,000)<br>3 = Low (1/100,000)<br>4 = Moderate (1/10,000)<br>5 = Moderate (1/2,000)<br>6 = Moderate (1/500)<br>7 = High (1/100)<br>8 = High (1/50)<br>9 = Very high (1/20)<br>10 = Very high (>1/10) | <Current improvement initiatives to remedy the failure mode with apparent effectiveness> | <Metrics or processes to detect failure mode with operational definitions> | 1 = Almost certain<br>2 = Very high<br>3 = High<br>4 = Moderate high<br>5 = Moderate<br>6 = Low<br>7 = Very low<br>8 = Remote<br>9 = Very remote<br>10 = Almost impossible | Sum:<br>Severity Score +<br>Occurrence Score +<br>Detection Score | <Actions recommended by team to prevent failure mode or to mitigate the effects> | <Accountable individual, division, department, or organization to complete recommended actions> | <Date actions to be completed> | <Actions taken to eliminate failure mode or mitigate effects> | <Date actions were completed> | | | | |

**Table 3-5** RPNs for falls with injury intervention

| Step | Description | Severity | Occurrence | Detection | RPN |
|------|-------------|----------|------------|-----------|-----|
| 1 | Awaken for morning bath; assist out of bed | 8 | 5 | 3 | 120 |
| 2 | Return to bed after morning bath | 8 | 2 | 2 | 32 |
| 3 | Breakfast served at bedside | 5 | 2 | 2 | 20 |
| 4 | Transport to/from physical therapy | 9 | 5 | 3 | 135 |
| 5 | Physical therapy (1 hour per day) | 9 | 6 | 2 | 108 |
| 6 | Lunch served at bedside | 5 | 2 | 2 | 20 |
| 7 | Afternoon free time | 9 | 7 | 6 | 378 |
| 8 | Dinner served in dining area | 7 | 4 | 4 | 112 |
| 9 | Evening meds, "tuck in" | 4 | 2 | 3 | 24 |
| 10 | Overnight | 8 | 5 | 7 | 280 |

# DELIVERABLES IN THE MEASURE PHASE

All of the tools that have been described are directed at achieving a set of deliverables for this phase that include:

- Data collection and analysis plan
  - Process metrics with operational definitions
  - Measurement system analysis
- Baseline performance—often summarized in calculation of process sigma

The ability of the team to proceed with the DMAIC process relies on timely and accurate information for these key factors.

## Data Collection and Analysis Plan

### Process Metrics with Operational Definitions

At this point in the Measure Phase, process maps are done and initial measurements have been performed that identify key process metrics. These measures fall into three categories:

- **Outcome measures**—metrics that demonstrate a change in the objective of the process improvement. For example, a project to improve diabetic eye exams could have an outcome measure "percent of patients with diabetic retinopathy." In some cases process and outcome measures can be difficult to differentiate. For example, if a project were to aim for improvement of use of beta-blocking drugs after MI, would the outcome be increased use of beta-blockers? Actually, most people would consider that metric to be a process measure and the reduction in post-MI recurrences and complications would be the outcome measure.

- **Process measures**—these measures are usually associated with a step in the process that is the target of an intervention. For example, the diabetic eye exam process measure could be "percent of diabetics with an annual eye exam." Other process measures for the diabetes eye exam project may be "percent of diabetics with telephone reminder contact" or "percent of diabetics with at least one annual visit to ophthalmologist." In general, the quality improvement approach assumes that process measures must improve to create any improvement in outcome measures. Most improvement projects will have several process measures.

- **Balancing measures**—these measures are often used as a way of determining how a change in one part of the system creates changes in other parts of the enterprise. In the diabetic eye exam project, for example, encouraging diabetics to undergo annual eye exams may cause a short tem increase in cost of care, but those costs should be balanced by savings from the costs of caring for the complications of diabetic retinopathy in the future. Thus, the project would measure not only costs of the current intervention, but also the cost savings over the period in which the effects of the intervention should be realized. In the case of diabetic eye exams, the cost savings will likely be realized as much as five years into the future through a decreased incidence of diabetic retinopathy and associated costs of care. Balancing measures may also be used to determine if another part of the enterprise has been detrimentally affected by an improvement, as well.

Operational definitions are clear explanations of the variable(s) to be measured for the metric. An operational definition identifies one or more specific observable conditions or events and then tells the observer how to measure the condition or event. Typically, variables and values may have more than one potential operational definition, and so each measure must be clearly defined before measurement begins.

Operational definitions must be valid (i.e., they must measure what they are supposed to measure). Additionally, operational definitions must be reliable; the results should be the same regardless of who performs the measurement or when the measurement is made. An example operational definition form for Average Length of Stay is shown in **Figure 3-16**.

---

HOSPITAL MEASURE INFORMATION FORM B:

Average Length of Stay

---

**Indicator Statement:** The overall average length of stay for all inpatient discharges per month

**Rationale for Selection**: Identifying the length of stay will promote an understanding of resource utilization required to care for patients served and may be correlated to medical errors. The length of stay (LOS) of hospitals patients mix can reveal the acuity level of the said population. As the length of stay for these patients increase, there are associated operational implications including increased system costs, resource utilization and appropriate alignment of resource allocation across the system. Additional stratification will be developed for this indicator to better identify the contributing factors for length of stay over the next 6 months, including data such as the patients place of residence, the number of procedures performed, etc.

**Type of Measure:** Process                **Measure Category:** Human Resources, Financial

---

**Numerator Statement:** Number of total inpatient discharge days per month
    **Numerator Description**
    **Included Populations:** All inpatients
    **Excluded Populations:** All outpatient services, outreach clinics or clinic visits
**Denominator Statement:** The total number of discharges per month for all inpatients
    **Denominator Description**
    **Included Populations:** All inpatients
    **Excluded Populations:** All outpatient services, outreach clinics or clinic visits
**Source of Measure:** Headquarters 3M Analytic Workstation system and/or the Shriners Hospitals for Children Information System
**Discharge Days:** The number of days that elapse between the patients day of admission and the patients day of discharge

---

Signature: _____ Date: _____

**FIGURE 3-16** Operational Definition form for Average Length of Stay

Operational definitions are clearly of great importance in formulating data collection and analysis strategies, since they define the data elements that need to be collected, as well as the format in which they are recorded so that the appropriate analysis may be performed.

## Measurement System Analysis

One of the key deliverables for the Measure Phase is a plan for data collection and analysis. The focus of data collection should be to gather data that helps to describe the problem, as well as uncovering any factors that provide clues about how, when, where, or in what circumstances the problem occurs or worsens. During planning, the team must not only determine what data to collect, but also ensure that the collection process is valid. The Six Sigma approach includes a process, called gauge repeatability and reproducibility (gauge R&R) that ensures that the collection (measurement) process is valid and that the act of collecting data does not distort the actual data values. The two parameters in this framework are:

- **Repeatability**—the variation in measurements taken by a single person or instrument on the same item, under the same conditions; for example, the same person weighing the same baby multiple times on the same scale will realize a certain amount of variation that must be accounted for in the measurement system.
- **Reproducibility**—the variation induced by different people or instruments doing the measurement (i.e., if multiple people are making the same measurement on the same item, how much difference is there between the measurements)?

Gauge R&R uses statistical methods to evaluate the amount of variability created by the measurement system itself. This variation is compared with the total variation in the measurement, and if the measurement methods add too much "noise," then the measurement approach may not be useful. Consider, for example, weight scales that are used in a medical office to measure children's weights at a well child checkup. Most of these scales are accurate to a level of a few grams, since a 30-gram variation in a 20 kilogram child is unlikely to indicate any problems. On the other hand, the scales used to weigh babies in the premature nursery must be accurate to much closer tolerances, since in a 1500-gram baby, a variation of 30 grams within a prescribed time frame can be an indicator of problems like a fluid deficit. Thus the scales in the premature nursery are built to achieve much higher accuracy and precision. Gauge R&R considers several factors that affect a measurement system:

- **Measuring instruments**—the gauge or measurement instrument and all associated equipment, housings, mountings, supports, fixtures, and other attachments. Included in this analysis is the ease of use, allowed variability in use of the machine (e.g., an office scale may allow a child to be clothed or unclothed, which will affect the weight), and other sources of "noise" in the measurement.
- **Human factors**—the training, capability, and discipline of the person using the instrument to follow the written or verbal instructions in use of the tool.
- **Test methods**—the methods used to test the instrument (e.g., how a scale is set to zero) as well as methods of collecting and recording data.
- **Tolerance levels**—the closeness a reference measurement is to the actual value of the reference specimen's true measure; for example, use of a reference weight to test the closeness of a scale's measurement to the "true" value. Although the tolerance may not directly affect the measurement, it does indicate an error correction factor that must be considered in the measurement system.
- **Measured items**—the item being measured must be appropriate for the instrument being used. For example, weighing a 40-kilogram adolescent on a baby scale makes no sense whatsoever and would probably break the scale!

Gauge R&R addresses the *precision* of a measurement system, or the reproducibility of a measurement. Accuracy is the closeness of the measurement to the true value, and gauge R&R is not designed to detect that type of measurement problem. The P/T ratio is sometimes used to express the level of reproducibility of a measurement process:

$$\frac{P}{T} = \frac{\text{Precision}}{\text{Total tolerance}}$$

This equation expresses the ratio of the precision of a measurement system to the total tolerance of the process of which it is a part. A low P/T ratio indicates that the impact of the measurement variation on the quality of the end result is small; on the other hand, if the P/T ratio is large, then the measurement system could contribute to an incorrect value for the end result. In general, a P/T ratio less than 0.1 indicates that the measurement system is sufficiently reliable, while a ratio over 0.3, the measurement system is likely not reliable enough to perform the measurement.

A Gauge R&R analysis is performed by using the measurement system on a known quantity and identifying as many sources of variation as possible. This phase of the evaluation is conducted before the measurement system is used in a live situation to ensure that the multiple potential sources of error are identified and mitigated. For example, when the pediatric office described above purchases a new scale, everyone using the scale may perform ten or twenty measurements of a standard weight to determine the range of the values, assessing the reasons causing variation in the measurements. Not only will this approach determine repeatability (i.e. variation caused by each person performing the weights), but it will also help capture reproducibility errors, since everyone using the instrument will be "tested". The results of these tests can then be analyzed statistically to determine the level of validity of the measurement system.

Performing a Gauge R&R analysis is particularly important in a six sigma project, since the tolerances are so small. To achieve a six sigma level of 3.4 defects per million opportunities (DPMO) requires a high level of precision in the measurement system, and so ensuring that the measurement system is valid prior to initiating an intervention is important to ensure that the results from the intervention are not just from measurement system "noise".

# BASELINE PERFORMANCE— CALCULATING PROCESS SIGMA

Six sigma performance connotes 3.4 DPMO, or a process that delivers output that meets customer specifications 99.9997% of the time. Although a laudable goal, most DMAIC projects in health care cannot achieve this level of quality without incurring substantial costs and making other tradeoffs. Process sigma is a useful measure, however, for a number of reasons. First, it is a single number that can be easily understood as an "index of performance" – the higher the sigma level, the better the performance level. Secondly, since it is based on customer Critical to Quality (CTQ) parameters for a particular process, it can be used generically between processes to assess how well each process is meeting the CTQ requirements. Thus, laboratory processes can be compared with patient throughput systems which can be compared with pharmacy accuracy systems using the process sigma levels. This ability is particularly important for managers who might use the process sigma levels as one factor to prioritize different projects for intervention. Finally, the process sigma is a useful metric for assessing overall process improvement as interventions are implemented, allowing an improvement team to simplify reports to senior managers to demonstrate the effects of improvement activities.

One widely used method of calculating the sigma level is by first calculating the DPMO and then looking up the sigma level in a table like that in Table 3.6.

**Table 3-6** DPMO – Sigma table

| DPMO | Sigma value | DPMO | Sigma value |
|---|---|---|---|
| 309,000 | 2.0 | 4,660 | 4.1 |
| 274,000 | 2.1 | 3,470 | 4.2 |
| 242,000 | 2.2 | 2,560 | 4.3 |
| 212,000 | 2.3 | 1,870 | 4.4 |
| 184,000 | 2.4 | 1,350 | 4.5 |
| 159,000 | 2.5 | 968 | 4.6 |
| 136,000 | 2.6 | 687 | 4.7 |
| 115,000 | 2.7 | 483 | 4.8 |
| 96,800 | 2.8 | 337 | 4.9 |
| 80,800 | 2.9 | 233 | 5.0 |
| 66,800 | 3.0 | 159 | 5.1 |
| 54,800 | 3.1 | 108 | 5.2 |
| 44,600 | 3.2 | 72 | 5.3 |
| 35,900 | 3.3 | 48 | 5.4 |
| 28,700 | 3.4 | 32 | 5.5 |
| 22,800 | 3.5 | 21 | 5.6 |
| 17,900 | 3.6 | 13 | 5.7 |
| 13,900 | 3.7 | 9 | 5.8 |
| 10,700 | 3.8 | 5 | 5.9 |
| 8,200 | 3.9 | 3.4 | 6.0 |
| 6,210 | 4.0 | | |

DPMO is calculated by first computing the number of defects per opportunity and then multiplying that number by 1 million:

$$DPO = \frac{\text{Number of defects}}{\text{Number of units} \times \text{Number of opportunities}}$$

$$DPMO = DPO \times 10^6$$

Once the DPMO value is known, the sigma value can be determined from the table.

---

## Example 3-4 Calculating Process Sigma

The pharmacy department at Perfection Clinic was concerned about its medication error rate and decided to calculate the sigma level for the medication delivery process, which primarily was focused on the work of the pharmacists within the department. They measured the number of reported errors daily for a month, which averaged 5 errors per day. The department filled an average of 1500 prescriptions per day, and each prescription was considered one unit. The DPMO calculation was performed as follows:

$$DPO = \frac{5 \text{ defects}}{1 \text{ units } \times 1500 \text{ opportunities}} = \frac{1}{300} DPO$$

$$DPMO = \frac{1}{300} \times 10^6 = 3{,}333$$

From Table 3.6, a DPMO of 3,333 coincides most closely with a sigma level of about 4.2.

---

# FINISHING THE MEASURE PHASE

At the end of the Measure phase, the project team should have a detailed process map, detailed baseline data, operational definitions for process metrics, CTCs and CTQs, a data collection and analysis plan, and a calculation of baseline process sigma. This information should provide team members with a clear understanding of the process steps and current level of performance. Armed with this data, the team can proceed to the Analyze Phase.

# FURTHER READING

Pyzdek T and Keller P, The Six Sigma Handbook, 2009, McGraw Hill, Columbus, OH.

Breyfogle F, Implementing Six Sigma: Smarter Solutions Using Statistical Methods: Second Edition, 2003, John Wiley and Sons, Hoboken, NJ.

Caldwell C, Brexler J, Gillem T, Lean-Six SIGMA for Healthcare: A Senior Leader Guide to Improving Cost and Throughput, 2005. ASQ Press, Milwaukee, WI.

# DISCUSSION QUESTIONS

1. What is the fundamental equation of six sigma? Explain what the terms mean.
2. How is a process map used during the Measure Phase? What types of process maps may be useful to teams during this phase?
3. Create a PERT chart for a process with which you are familiar using the format defined in Figure 3-1.
4. Create a deployment flowchart for a process with which you are familiar using the format in Figure 3-4.
5. Work with two or three others to complete a prioritization matrix based on a brainstorming exercise on improving a common process like deciding on a computer to purchase.
6. What is process cycle efficiency? How can it be used to assess a process?
7. How is time value analysis used to focus the team on opportunities for improvement? Perform a TVA on your typical workday.
8. Describe the basis for the Pareto chart. Create a Pareto chart in Excel using the following data table:

| Cause | Effect |
|---|---|
| 1 | 18 |
| 2 | 92 |
| 3 | 31 |
| 4 | 53 |
| 5 | 29 |

9. How is a run chart used to analyze trend data? What is runs analysis? How does a runs analysis help evaluate process performance and variation?

10. How does a control chart differ from a run chart? Can runs analysis be applied to a control chart? Explain how a control chart is used to identify levels of variation and process performance.
11. What is the difference between attributes data and continuous data? How does that difference relate to selection of a control chart?
12. Describe the FMECA. What is the criticality score and risk priority number? How are these values used in FMECA?
13. What are the three types of measures for any process? Define and give examples of each.
14. What is an operational definition? Why is an operational definition important to a quality improvement data gathering process?
15. Describe gauge R&R. How is gauge R&R used in the Measure Phase? What does gauge R&R NOT assess?

# CHAPTER 4

# Analyze Phase Tools

*"A good catchword can obscure analysis for fifty years."*

—Wendell Willkie

*"Definition of a Statistician: A man who believes figures don't lie, but admits that under analysis some of them won't stand up either."*

—Evan Esar

*"Familiar things happen, and mankind does not bother about them. It requires a very unusual mind to undertake the analysis of the obvious."*

—Alfred North Whitehead

*"Get the habit of analysis—analysis will in time enable synthesis to become your habit of mind."*

—Frank Lloyd Wright

## THE ESSENCE OF THE ANALYZE PHASE

The Measure and Analyze phases make the Six Sigma approach unique. Few quality improvement approaches delve into the analytic dimension of performance like the Six Sigma process does during these two phases. The Analyze Phase is directed at developing hypotheses regarding the causes of

**111**

poor performance, and then validating the hypotheses using the data that has been collected during the Define and Measure phases. The focus that emanates from this phase helps direct the improvement initiatives during the next phase in a way that is concentrated on leveraging efforts to gain the greatest possible change at the lowest possible cost.

# ELEMENTS OF THE ANALYZE PHASE

During the Analyze Phase, the value of the Six Sigma Black Belt becomes acutely apparent. The application of the scientific method involves development of a hypothesis, determining appropriate analytic approaches for testing the hypothesis, and then coming to conclusions that will help drive the Improve Phase. Tools used in this phase include some that have been described before:

- 5 Whys analysis (Root Cause Analysis)
- Cause and effect diagram
- Affinity diagram—described in Chapter 2
- Control charts—described in Chapter 3
- Flow diagrams—described in Chapters 2 and 3
- Pareto charts—described in Chapter 3
- Correlation analysis
- Hypothesis testing
- Analysis of Variance (ANOVA)
- Regression analysis and scatter plots
- Brainstorming—described in Chapter 2

During the Measure Phase the baseline performance of the process has been defined through collection and collation of data that now can be prioritized using the techniques of the Analyze Phase. Using tools like regression analysis it is possible to hone in on the source of the problem and determine the level of influence that each underlying cause exerts on the target outcome. The key to this phase, which is unique to the Six Sigma approach, is application of the scientific approach (hypothesis testing) to improving the performance of a process. There are several benefits of this approach:

- Improved reliability of the inferences made about underlying causes of a problem. If the team selects appropriate causative factors and metrics during the Measure Phase, the analyses can place a statistically tested level of importance to each of these factors. The increased reliability that results from this information leads to significant benefits in subsequent phases.

- The analytic approach developed during this phase is applied to determining if interventions designed in the Improve Phase to assess the effect of the interventions, and sometimes even in the Control Phase for ongoing monitoring of the process. Quantitative monitoring of the process is often reassuring to process owners, since it provides an objective way to ensure process performance.

- The information that emanates from the Analyze Phase directs improvement efforts in a way that enhances the return on the investment that a team makes in improvement initiatives. By using these data, the team can find the most influential factor that is affecting performance and concentrate efforts on that item to leverage the initiative to gain the biggest effect possible.

- In health care, there is a tendency to perform "knee jerk" analyses of root causes that often ignores important factors and misdirects improvement efforts, leading to failed improvement projects and loss of confidence in the quality improvement approach. Scientifically trained professionals like physicians and nurses find typical improvement approaches based just on brainstorming or other nondata-centric root cause identification methods less than compelling, but the use of the scientific method in Six Sigma, highlighted in the Analyze Phase, often helps validate the approach to such skeptics.

These benefits help quality improvement staff to justify the investments in time and resources to support change and achieve improvements.

## Root Cause Analysis (RCA)

Root Cause Analysis has grown to be a much more sophisticated approach over the past several years. Starting decades earlier as the "5 Whys," RCA has evolved into a highly effective analytic approach that dives deeply into a process to uncover multiple layers of causation. One common concept of the way that errors are propagated throughout a system to create an unfavorable outcome is the "swiss cheese model," as illustrated in **Figure 4-1**.

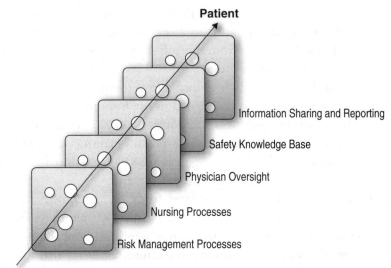

Data from: Agency for Healthcare Research and Quality, Patient Safety Network, accessed at http://www.psnet.ahrq.gov/glossary.aspx?indexLetter=S

**FIGURE 4-1** Swiss cheese model of error propagation

This model demonstrates that an error is usually not due to failures with just one system or one person, but rather shows that multiple systems and processes usually fail to produce an error. Thus, a one-dimensional review of the failure will miss many of the underlying problems in numerous processes that led to the error. Sophisticated systems, like the TapRooT system designed by Systems Improvement, Inc., have been designed to track down these issues, using principles of human performance and equipment reliability that enhance the identification of underlying causes. Although the RCA may be performed manually, use of a software system can improve success and increase the likelihood that all important root causes are identified.

The 5 Whys constitute the older, simpler approach pioneered as part of the Toyota Production System. Application of the 5 Whys involves taking any problem and asking, "Why did this happen? What caused this problem?" By repeatedly asking the question "Why?" it is possible to gradually peel away layers of causes to uncover the root cause of a problem. Each "Why" leads to a subsequent question that finally results in root cause identification. In many cases the five "Whys" are sufficient, but sometimes, the technique will continue beyond that level as new issues are recognized.

### Procedure for RCA

The procedure for RCA follows a specific sequence:

1. Define the issue to be evaluated
2. Gather data relating to the issue
3. Apply the 5 Whys to hone in on the root cause of the problem
4. Brainstorm corrective action(s) that may be expected to remedy the root causes
   - Within the control of the team
   - Meet goals and objectives
   - Do not cause other problems elsewhere in the system
5. Implement the recommendations and measure the effects using metrics developed along with the corrective action(s)

The basic elements of RCA are listed in **Table 4-1**. These issues can be used to start tracking down root causes by organizing the inquiries into specific categories and beginning to ask specific questions regarding potential causes.

An example of the 5 Whys analysis is included in **Example 4-1**. The 5 Whys may be used in relatively straightforward circumstances, but for most problems that create a significant problem for the organization, a formal RCA must be conducted supported by software programs that ensure consideration of all potential underlying reasons. In healthcare systems that have significant errors that risk patient safety, the stakes are too high to do an inadequate RCA.

### Tips and Tricks

1. RCA involves brainstorming or one of its variants, and so every effort must be made to involve as many stakeholders in these reviews as possible. However, the team performing the RCA should be relatively small and focused with expertise in conducting these analyses.
2. In many industries, RCAs are called "investigations." Practical use of the RCA approach in health care suggests that the word "investigation" might be perceived as threatening. Many healthcare organizations have adopted the terminology "assessment" or "review" to avoid the negative connotation of "investigation."

**Table 4-1** Root cause analysis factors

| Category | Elements | Example |
|---|---|---|
| Materials | • Defective raw material<br>• Wrong material<br>• Unavailability of material | • Lack of appropriate sized endotracheal tube during a resuscitation |
| Manpower | • Inadequate physical capability<br>• Lack of training<br>• Stress from job or personal factors<br>• Lack of motivation | • Floating nurse in hospital not trained for a specialty floor |
| Machine/ equipment | • Incorrect equipment or tools<br>• Lack of maintenance or design<br>• Unavailability of proper tool or equipment<br>• Defective equipment | • Ventilator broken when needed in ICU |
| Environment | • Disorderly environment or workflow<br>• Excessive physical demands<br>• Inadequate cleaning<br>• Lack of safeguards | • Moving patient from stretcher to bed without assistance |
| Management | • No supervision or poor oversight<br>• Lack of attention<br>• Lack of defined process | • Patient cardiac alarm not attended |
| Methods | • Lack of defined procedures<br>• Failure to follow defined procedures<br>• Poor communication | • Workarounds for Computerized Physician Order Entry |
| Management system | • Lack of training<br>• Lack of employee involvement in planning or implementation<br>• Lack of hazard recognition<br>• Failure to eliminate hazards | • Managers implement a new process for medication administration without working with staff |

3. RCA frequently produces surprising results when done properly. Although some problems may seem to have self-evident solutions, an effective RCA will identify many other issues with requirements for more system-based solutions. Thus, if there is any doubt about whether to perform a full RCA, it is better to proceed with the analysis.

# Example 4-1 The 5 Whys applied to a problem

Although RCA is usually applied to problems with systems, it also can be used to identify the underlying causes of any problem. The nursing staff on the oncology unit noticed that the rate of IV infiltrations had increased over the past four weeks. The number of IV restarts had doubled in that time period, so they applied RCA's 5 Whys to the problem:

1. Why are the IV lines infiltrating?—The tubing seems to be moving excessively when the patient moves.
2. Why does the tubing move when the patient moves?—The tubing seems to slip with movement of the IV site (e.g., the arm).
3. Why does the tubing slip with movement of the IV site?—The tape that is holding the plastic tube allows the tubing to slide between pieces of tape.
4. Why does the tape allow the tubing to slip?—The adhesive on the tape is not holding the tubing.
5. Why is the adhesive not holding the tubing?—Central Supply states that they started buying tape from a different vendor (lowest bidder) last month.

The team decided to go back to the original brand of tape, and the problem was resolved.

## Cause and Effect (C & E) Diagram

Kaoru Ishikawa is credited with developing the cause and effect diagram, which has become a standard tool of performance improvement. The Ishikawa diagram, also called the "Fishbone diagram," succinctly summarizes multiple causes and relates them to one major effect, as shown in **Figure 4-2**.

The main branches of the tree in Figure 4.2 represent the issues that the team identified as primary causes of the effect (low immunization rates), and each of the stems on the branches indicate the contributory factors that created each of the causes. Each of the stems should be subdivided until a measurable underlying cause is found. So, for example, the cost branch has a stem labeled "Insurance"; that stem may be further subdivided into other elements (e.g., "Commercial" and "Medicaid") and each of those components may be subdivided further until a measurable issue is defined.

The main branches can be labeled with any categories the team deems useful, but most often they have fairly standard designations. For manufacturing applications of the approach, the most common categories are

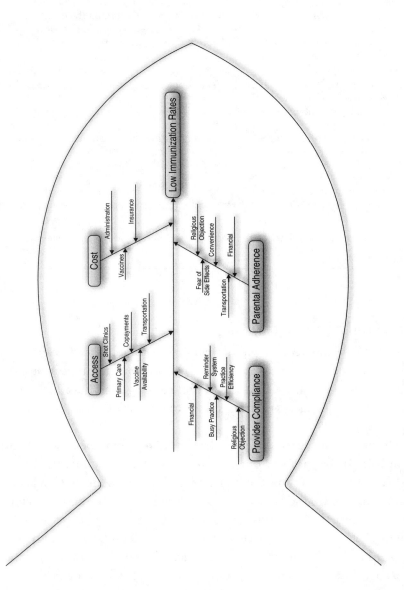

**FIGURE 4-2** Ishikawa Diagram for low immunization rates

Manpower, Methods, Materials, and Machinery, while service industries like health care typically use Equipment, Policies, Procedures, and People. If the team is having trouble deciding on the branches, it is often helpful to start with one of these classification schemes as a way of creating focus on the issues. The affinity diagram (Chapter 2) is one way of discovering a set of categories for the Ishikawa diagram, and the headers on the affinity diagram can be used as the categories in the cause and effect diagram.

### Procedure for Cause and Effect Diagram

Typically, the C&E diagram is created on a flipchart or whiteboard, but Visio® is a useful software program to create and edit these diagrams.

1. Agree on a problem issue (effect) and record it at the center right of the flipchart or whiteboard. Draw a box around the issue statement, and then draw a horizontal arrow pointing into the box.
2. Work with the team to brainstorm the major categories of causes of the issue, using the following generic categories if more specific categories cannot be identified.
   - Methods
   - Machines (equipment)
   - People (workforce)
   - Materials
   - Measurement
   - Environment
3. Distribute the category descriptions above and below the horizontal line and connect the descriptions to the horizontal arrow with arrows pointing to the horizontal line.
4. For each branch, brainstorm all the possible causes of the problem and add each cause to the diagram along the category arrows with additional arrows pointing into the category arrow. The same cause may be used for multiple branches if it is related to more than one category.
5. When all the ideas have been recorded the group can focus attention on the sparsest branches to determine if more causes might be present. After all potential causes have been entered on the chart, the team must prioritize the categories using a technique like Pareto analysis.

**Tips and Tricks**

1. The brainstorming sessions for cause and effect diagrams may produce duplicate or similar ideas, and the team may need to use a list reduction technique like multivoting to make the list of causes more manageable.

2. Even with a robust Ishikawa diagram, the team will need to prioritize categories for efficient and effective interventions. Although brainstorming might be one approach to consider, use of data can make the prioritization more effective. Pareto analysis is one way to establish priorities, but other methods discussed later in this chapter, like multiple regression, might be even more effective.

3. The cause and effect diagram is one of the best graphics to use when presenting a complex problem to senior managers. A relatively large amount of information can be concisely placed in an easy to understand diagram, leading to the popularity of the Ishikawa diagram.

## *Statistical Methods of Establishing Relationships*

Six Sigma precision depends on establishing relationships between dependent (outcome) variables and independent (process) variables. For example, a surgical site infection (SSI) is a detrimental outcome measure represented by a dependent variable that might be coded as "Yes" if an infection occurs and "No" if an infection does not occur within the defined postoperative period. An improvement team is interested in which factors might be related to the presence of an SSI, and so the team may brainstorm a number of factors that they think might be at fault, for example:

- Lack of a sterile field
- Contaminated instruments
- Surgery performed in Operating Room 5
- "Dirty wound" preoperatively
- Specific surgeon
- Type of procedure (e.g., abdominal, thoracic, genitourinary)
- Presence of complications (e.g., lung disease, anemia, heart disease)
- Lack of preoperative antibiotics

The question arises, however, "how important is each one of the variables?" The question is significant, since the team's efforts and resources can be directed at the most significant variables to start, rather than taking a "shotgun" approach and likely misdirecting those efforts. A number of tools help solve this problem. This section is not meant to be a statistics course, but rather provide the basis for "statistical thinking" (i.e., the ability to know what statistical tests might be helpful in a particular situation). Myriad statistical tests are available, and a Six Sigma Black Belt is trained in the application of the various methods. Additionally, these tests are also discussed in more depth in *Advanced Performance Improvement in Health Care: Principles and Methods* by Lighter. The tests that will be discussed here include:

- Pearson correlation coefficient
- Analysis of variance (ANOVA)
- Linear regression
- Multiple regression
- Chi square analysis

These techniques are the most commonly used in Lean Six Sigma and basic knowledge of their application and the information they provide can help enrich the value of a project.

### Pearson Correlation Coefficient

The Pearson correlation coefficient (sometimes called the Pearson moment correlation coefficient), represented by "r," helps understand the level and direction of a relationship between two variables. In LSS, this value is used to determine if any relationship exists between two observed data values or two seemingly random variables. The Pearson r can vary from –1 to +1 and is interpreted as follows:

- –1 = an inverse relationship exists between the two variables (i.e., as one variable increases, the other variable will decrease)
- 0 = no relationship exists between the variables
- +1 = a direct relationship exists between the two variables (i.e., as one variable increases, the other variable increases)

One way of examining the relationship is to draw a scatterplot of the two variables as shown in **Figure 4-3**, which graphs the data in **Table 4-2** that was obtained from measurements taken by a managed care organization

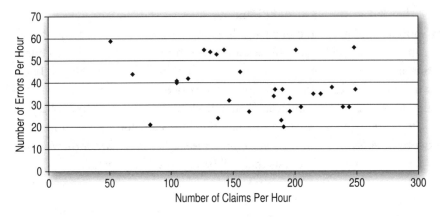

**FIGURE 4-3** Scatterplot

that collected the number of claims processed per hour in a department and related it to the number of errors in processing by the department. The scatterplot does not seem to demonstrate much of a relationship, and so further analysis using a Pearson correlation coefficient was performed on the data set, yielding a Pearson r-value of –0.29 that indicates an inverse relationship that is relatively weak. The scatterplot graphically indicates the weak relationship, but the Pearson r confirms it and provides a little extra information that the relationship is negative. Frequently, the Pearson's r will only hint at a relationship and indicate a need for further study.

The difference between an association and causation is important to understand. Although the Pearson r may show that two variables are related, the nature of the relationship cannot be inferred. In other words, simply demonstrating a relationship between two variables does not allow one to conclude that one variable "causes" the change in the other variable. For example, the relationship between chronic disease and depression may show a rather strong correlation, but it is not possible to determine if depression causes chronic disease or if the chronic disease causes patients to be depressed. Some causal relationships may be posited however, such as the relationship between parental height and that of their children. Since a strong relationship can be shown via a correlation statistic like the Pearson r, the inference can be made that parental height is a causative factor for their children's stature. However, other factors also may be at work, so the relationship will doubtless not be a "perfect" Pearson's r of 1.

**Table 4-2** Data collected for scatterplot: Number of claims per hour vs. number of errors per hour

| Number of claims/hour | Number of errors/hour |
|:---:|:---:|
| 230 | 38 |
| 190 | 37 |
| 244 | 29 |
| 215 | 35 |
| 183 | 34 |
| 143 | 55 |
| 105 | 41 |
| 69 | 44 |
| 138 | 24 |
| 147 | 32 |
| 201 | 55 |
| 248 | 56 |
| 191 | 20 |
| 114 | 42 |
| 163 | 27 |
| 156 | 45 |
| 137 | 53 |
| 249 | 37 |
| 196 | 27 |
| 132 | 54 |
| 221 | 35 |
| 105 | 40 |
| 184 | 37 |
| 205 | 29 |
| 189 | 23 |
| 239 | 29 |
| 69 | 44 |
| 51 | 59 |
| 83 | 21 |
| 196 | 33 |
| 127 | 55 |

Correlations are useful because they can define a predictive relationship that is useful for performance improvement. For example, a physician's office may be able to determine that the number of visits increases during the first quarter of each year due to respiratory diseases and then the number decreases in the second quarter as the respiratory illness cycle wanes. That relationship allows the office manager to have more staff available during the winter months and then reduce the staff in the spring and early summer. This "time of year" correlation suggests that winter causes more visits, when in fact it is the respiratory diseases that become prevalent during winter that are the actual cause. Thus, even a strong relationship may need to be further dissected to find the true underlying cause.

Importantly, the Pearson r detects only linear relationships between two variables (i.e., a relationship that can be graphed as a line on a scatterplot). For nonlinear relationships, other correlation coefficients have been developed; however, in most situations in the performance improvement world, the linear relationship is most common. The correlation coefficient is called a summary statistic and cannot replace examination of the data. For example, the data in Table 4-2 and the associated scatterplot provide a fair amount of information that indicates a relatively weak relationship, which is then verified by the Pearson's r. However, the Pearson's r helps with an understanding of the direction and magnitude of the relationship.

### Procedure for the Pearson Correlation Coefficient

Although the Pearson correlation coefficient can be calculated from its formula, the best way to perform the test is to use Microsoft Excel's® PEARSON function. The PEARSON function calculates the r statistic that assesses the correlation between two arrays (columns or rows) of data in a spreadsheet. The procedure is as follows:

1. Arrange the two data sets of interest in rows or columns such as that in Table 4-2.
2. Select an open cell and enter: =PEARSON(array 1, array 2), where array 1 is the range of the first group of cells and array 2 is the range of the second group of cells.
3. The cell will then contain the Pearson r statistic.

## Tips and Tricks

1. The Pearson r suggests a relationship between two data arrays, but causality must be established in other ways (e.g., through specific experiments that control for other factors to isolate the effect of the independent variable of interest). Design of experiments (DOE) will be discussed in more detail in Chapter 5.
2. This statistic assumes a linear relationship between two variables. Although most relationships can fit a linear pattern, in some cases, such as that in the scatterplot in **Figure 4-4**, the pattern is distinctly not linear. In those cases, the Pearson r is not appropriate and other correlation statistics should be used.
3. The square of the Pearson correlation coefficient is $r^2$ is known as the coefficient of determination and represents the "magnitude" of the relationship between the two variables, stated statistically as the "proportion of common variation in the two variables." The $r^2$ value helps to better understand the correlation between variables, with higher values indicating that the two variables tend to move together, thus strengthening the argument that the two variables are correlated.

## *Hypothesis Testing*

When improvement teams want to try interventions on a population, it is usually difficult and expensive to perform initiatives on the entire population.

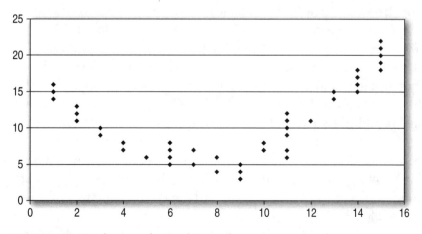

**FIGURE 4-4** Nonlinear relationship evident on a scatterplot

In most cases, the team will perform a pilot project on a sample of the population, using a matched sample that does not receive the intervention as a control group. With a simple two-factor analysis such as this, a simple t-test can be used to determine if the intervention had an effect. The statistical way of determining if the intervention was effective is a little unusual—it is called "rejecting the null hypothesis." The null hypothesis is usually stated as:

- **$H_0$: There is no difference between the treatment group and the control group after the treatment has been rendered.**

The null hypothesis implies that there is an alternative hypothesis, which is the opposite of the null:

- **$H_1$: There is a difference between the treatment group and the control group after the treatment has been rendered.**

The null hypothesis typically compares sample or population means. In order to ensure that the comparison is valid, a statistical test is applied to the data collected during an experiment with measurements before and after an intervention or treatment. Statistical tests can provide an assessment of the validity of the null hypothesis so that it can be either accepted or rejected. However, since the null hypothesis most often uses sample data, the test makes an assumption that the sample data represents the population from which it is obtained. This assumption is associated with two types of potential errors: Type I ($\alpha$) error and Type II ($\beta$) error. A Type I error occurs when the null hypothesis is rejected incorrectly, and this error is used to determine the level of confidence ($1 - \alpha$) in the conclusion made from the hypothesis test. For example, for a confidence level (p) of 0.05, the alpha risk must be 0.95. A Type II error occurs when the null hypothesis is accepted incorrectly (i.e., the null hypothesis should be rejected, but is not). This type of error is often called the consumer's risk because an effective intervention or treatment is incorrectly interpreted as ineffective. Many people find it easiest to remember that a Type I error connotes a false positive result, while a Type II error indicates a false negative result.

These errors are key to understanding hypothesis testing. Most statistical tests of the null hypothesis focus on the $\alpha$ error (i.e., rejection of a true null hypothesis). The $\alpha$ error denotes the level of confidence, or p-value, which is used to determine the critical value of the test statistic. Any test statistic is based on a particular statistical distribution; for example, the t-test is based on the t-distribution, as shown in **Figure 4-5**. The figure shows that the t-distribution probability density function looks like a normal distribution, but it is designed for sample sizes less than 30 data points. The graph is sometimes also represented as a table in which individual values of t can be found, but for most situations, using a program like Excel to find the t-value and the associated confidence level for comparison with the target confidence level is much easier.

If the null hypothesis takes the form "$H_0$: The means are the same," then the t-test that is applied is known as a two-tailed test, since rejection of the null hypothesis can occur if one mean is either greater than or less than the other mean. On the other hand, if the null hypothesis states "$H_0$: one mean is greater than the other mean" or "$H_0$: one mean is less than the other mean," then the t-test that is applied is a one-tailed test, since rejection of the null hypothesis occurs if only one condition is met, and the probability for $\alpha$ will be tested using only one tail (or end) of the distribution.

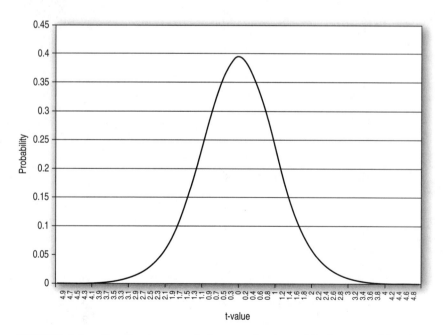

**FIGURE 4-5** t-distribution graph for sample size = 20, degrees of freedom = 19

### Procedure for t-Test

1. Determine the type of t-test to be used—one tail or two tail—based on the null hypothesis.
2. Using Microsoft Excel, put the baseline data collected in one column and the data collected following the intervention in an adjacent column as shown in **Table 4-3**.
3. In a separate cell, enter the t-test function using the first data column as array 1, the second data column as array 2, and then select the number of tails based on the null hypothesis in step 1. The final

**Table 4-3** Example data for two-tailed t-test with t-probability

| Subject number | Before | After |
|:---:|:---:|:---:|
| 1 | 2 | 8 |
| 2 | 2 | 3 |
| 3 | 4 | 8 |
| 4 | 4 | 5 |
| 5 | 4 | 7 |
| 6 | 1 | 9 |
| 7 | 1 | 1 |
| 8 | 4 | 5 |
| 9 | 4 | 3 |
| 10 | 3 | 1 |
| 11 | 4 | 9 |
| 12 | 5 | 2 |
| 13 | 5 | 3 |
| 14 | 3 | 10 |
| 15 | 5 | 1 |
| 16 | 1 | 2 |
| 17 | 1 | 4 |
| 18 | 5 | 6 |
| 19 | 2 | 10 |
| 20 | 1 | 4 |
| 21 | 4 | 9 |
| t-probability | | 0.007788 |

selection for the t-test function, the type, indicates the type of data in the analysis. The three selections depend on the nature of the data:

   a. Value = 1—paired data, which compares means on the same or related subject over time or in differing circumstances (e.g., for subjects in a treatment protocol).

   b. Value = 2—two samples with equal variance, which compares means between samples from two normally distributed populations that have equal variance

   c. Value = 3—two samples with unequal variance compares means between samples from two normally distributed populations that have different variance values.

4. Compare the p-value obtained from the t-test function with the selected $\alpha$ value. For example, if the $\alpha$ value is 0.05, then any p-value that is less than 0.05 indicates that the null hypothesis can be rejected and the alternative hypothesis accepted.

The analysis for a two-tailed test is similar, except that the alternative hypothesis, $H_a$, is defined as satisfying more than one condition (i.e., $H_a$: mean 1 $\neq$ mean 2). In this situation, mean 1 can be greater than mean 2 or less than mean 2, so the $\alpha$ error must be distributed between two possibilities. The risk of each error (mean 1 > mean 2 and mean 1 < mean 2) becomes $\alpha/2$ or 0.025, even though the total $\alpha$ remains 0.05. In terms of the t-probability distribution shown in **Figures 4-6** and **4-7**, which show the two types of tests, the two-tailed test places half the risk at each end of the probability curve, while the one tailed test places all of the risk at one end.

The reason that the t-test is divided into one- and two-tailed versions is that the t-value to meet to exceed the desired $\alpha$ risk for the one-tailed version is greater than that for the two-tailed version (half the risk in each tail moves the threshold further out on the curve). A one-tailed test can thus be satisfied with a much lower difference between two values. However, using a one-tailed test also means that a direction for the relationship must be chosen pre-hoc as shown in Figure 4-6. Thus, if the t-value has a sign that is opposite that chosen for the hypothesized relationship, it will be outside the threshold and require acceptance of the null hypothesis that the two parameters being studied are the same. On the other hand, the t-value in a two-tailed test can be either positive or negative, which can be an advantage in many studies where the direction of the difference may not be known prior to performing a study. In most situations, it is enough to know that two values are not equal, allowing the use of a two-tailed t-test.

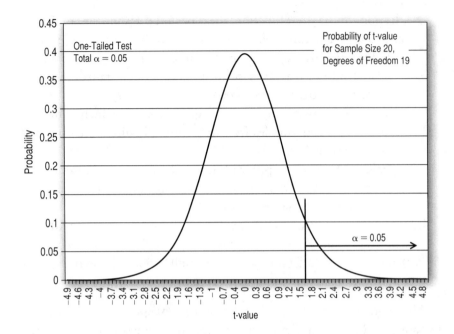

**FIGURE 4-6** One-tailed t-test distribution

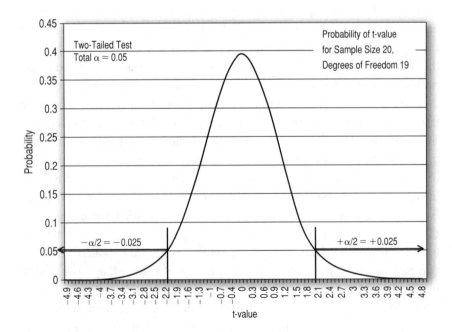

**FIGURE 4-7** Two-tailed t-test distribution

## Example 4-2 Use of a t-test for comparing samples

The administrator at a community hospital conducted a regular survey in the emergency department regarding patient satisfaction to determine if patients were satisfied with waiting time. The three-question survey used a Likert scale of 1–10, with 1 being very dissatisfied and 10 being very satisfied, and the average of the three questions was reported for each patient. The data in Table 4-3 provides the scores for a randomly selected sample of 21 patients before and after an intervention to reduce waiting times, with the average score reported by subject before and after the intervention. The administrator wanted to determine if the intervention had an effect, and he was not sure whether the intervention would have a positive or negative effect. Thus, the null and alternative hypotheses were:

- $H_0$: The intervention had no effect (the mean satisfaction is the same before and after the intervention)
- $H_a$: The intervention changed patient satisfaction (the mean satisfaction is either greater or worse after the intervention

The confidence level desired by the team was 95%, and so a p-value less than or equal to 0.05 would allow the team to reject the null hypothesis and accept the alternative hypothesis. A two-tailed t-test was applied to the data to determine the effect, and the p-value obtained is 0.007788 (rounded to 0.008), which is less than the p-value required to reject the null. Thus, the administrator concluded that the intervention had an effect.

The t-test is one of the most useful statistical tools used during the Analyze Phase, since it can provide direction to the improvement team by identifying relationships that are significant, as well as determining the level of confidence in the relationship. Additionally, the t-test can be used for pilot studies to determine if an intervention may have potential for wider dissemination, as shown in **Example 4-2**.

### Confidence Interval

A common task for improvement teams is trying to estimate a population value from sample data. Since a sample is taken from a population, it is assumed to represent the population, if the sample is chosen randomly, from the entire population. In practice, a truly random sample is difficult to attain. Some element of selection bias may enter into sample selection, making the sample only an approximation of the true population.

In those cases, the sample mean is an estimate of the population mean, and based on the sample size, the population standard deviation, and the level of confidence needed for the estimate (i.e., the $\alpha$ risk), a range for the mean can be determined. This range is called the confidence interval, and it defines a range in which the mean is centered. The formula for the confidence interval uses the population standard deviation ($\sigma$), the sample size, and the confidence level ($\alpha$) to calculate the interval on either side of the mean:

$$CI = Z_{\alpha/2} * \frac{\sigma}{\sqrt{n}}$$

CI = confidence interval

$Z_{\alpha/2}$ = the Z value from the standard normal distribution for the desired CI level for a two tailed test

$\sigma$= population standard deviation

n = sample size

---

## Example 4-3 Confidence interval for a population mean

A sample of 50 subjects is selected from a population to measure heights and predict the mean height of the population. The population is known to have a standard deviation of 10 cm for height, and the study requires a 95% level of confidence in the estimate of the mean. The mean height of the sample is determined to be 167.6 cm. The confidence interval is calculated as follows:

$$CI = Z_{\alpha/2} * \frac{\sigma}{\sqrt{n}} = 1.96 * \frac{10\,\text{cm}}{\sqrt{50}} = \frac{19.6}{7.1} = 2.8$$

The population mean is thus 167.6 + 2.8 cm (i.e., the population mean is predicted to be between 164.8 cm and 170.4 cm with a 95% level of confidence).

---

If a sample size less than 30 is used for the measurement, then the t-distribution table would be used. For example, if only 20 subjects were measured in **Example 4-3**, then $t_{\alpha/2}$ would be used in the equation rather than $Z_{\alpha/2}$, which would change the 1.96 value to 2.09 (the t-value for $\alpha = 0.05$ and $(20 - 1)$ degrees of freedom), making the CI = 2.9, and the range for the population mean widens to 164.7 – 170.5 cm.

Microsoft Excel® has built-in functions for the confidence interval: CONFIDENCE.NORM and CONFIDENCE.T. The CONFIDENCE. NORM function is used when the sample size (n) is greater than or equal to 30, and CONFIDENCE.T is used when the sample size is less than 30.

### Procedure for Confidence Interval for the Mean Using Excel

1. Determine the population standard deviation, if possible. If the population standard deviation is not available, it can be estimated by the sample standard error of the mean, which is calculated from the sample data.
2. Determine the sample size (n) and confidence level desired (often 95%, which is an $\alpha$ of 0.05).
3. Enter one of the CI formulas into an Excel cell based on sample size and enter the required parameters (desired $\alpha$ level, population $\sigma$, sample size n).
4. The resulting value is the CI on each side of the mean. So if a value of 2 is obtained from the calculation, the resulting interval around the mean ( $\overline{X}$ )would be:

$$\overline{X} \pm 2$$

The confidence interval is important to assess the reliability of the estimate. If the CI is large, i.e. the interval is wide, then the estimate is less reliable.

# ANALYSIS OF VARIANCE (ANOVA)

Analysis of variance (ANOVA) is used to test hypotheses about differences between two or more means, which allows more complex experiments using multiple variables to be performed. When there are more than two means to be compared, the t-test becomes unwieldy, and use of the t-test for multiple comparisons within the same intervention can lead to an artificially higher Type I error rate. ANOVA can be used to test for significant differences among several means without increasing the $\alpha$ risk. This statistical approach is most useful in those situations in which several groups have measurements done on one or more variables. For example, an improvement project may be designed to understand if differences exist between groups of patients (e.g. age stratified) on a satisfaction survey of hospital service.

As one might expect, the large variety of combinations of improvement interventions (think of them as "experiments") have led to multiple forms of ANOVA. The different types of ANOVA reflect the different experimental designs and situations for which they have been developed, and a list of several methods of ANOVA can be found in Table 4-4.

Most performance improvement projects involve single- or two-factor ANOVA, and the use of ANOVA depends on a thorough understanding of the data set and the hypothesis being tested, which typically falls within the scope of the Six Sigma Black Belt or a statistician.

ANOVA is a special case of multiple regression where the independent (x) variables are the categories, or factors. Each value of a factor is referred to as a level; so for example, three different drug doses in a medication efficacy study would indicate that the drug is the factor and the three different dosages are the levels, making this design a single factor, three level study. The dependent (Y), or outcome, variable in the relationship consists of the experimental values obtained as the drug is tested at the three doses. Although some ANOVA models can be very complex and need a Black Belt or statistician to do the analysis, many experimental models with only one or two factors can be performed using Microsoft Excel with a statistical add-in like QI Macros®.

**Table 4-4** ANOVA variants

| ANOVA type | Brief description |
| --- | --- |
| One way | One factor, fixed effects |
| Two way | Two factors, randomized blocks |
| Two way with repeated observations | Two factors, randomized block |
| Fully nested | Hierarchical factors |
| Latin square | One primary and two secondary factors |
| Crossover | Two factors, fixed effects, treatment crossover |
| Kruskal-Wallis | Nonparametric one way |
| Friedman | Nonparametric two way |
| Homogeneity of variance | Examine the ANOVA assumption of equal variance |
| Shapiro-Wilk W | Examine the ANOVA assumption of normality |
| Agreement | Examine agreement of two or more samples |

# Example 4-4 Analysis of Variance for interventions to improve patient satisfaction

Another day had passed at the New Wave Clinic, and the staff has continued to field complaints from patients regarding wait times, particular at the beginning of the patient encounter. Analyzing the processes of care, the team discovered that there were four steps during the process where problems caused delays in patient flow. The clinic manager pulled together a team of staff members to design potential interventions to improve patient wait times and thus satisfaction. The teams examined satisfaction data and came up with four potential interventions for the patient flow process. To determine which of the four interventions had the greatest potential for changing the waiting time, the team performed a pilot study over 2 months in four different randomly selected groups of patients seen in the clinic. Each group went through the process that differed only in the improvement intervention applied, identified as Interventions 1, 2, 3, and 4, and the waiting time was measured for a random sample of patients in each group. The waiting time data are reported in Table 4-5 and the results of a single factor ANOVA are shown in Table 4-6.

**Table 4-5** Data for pilot study of patient waiting times

|  | Baseline | Intervention 1 | Intervention 2 | Intervention 3 | Intervention 4 |
|---|---|---|---|---|---|
|  | 38.0 | 39.0 | 37.0 | 35.0 | 32.0 |
|  | 37.0 | 36.0 | 32.0 | 33.0 | 34.0 |
|  | 37.0 | 38.0 | 35.0 | 38.0 | 36.0 |
|  | 38.0 | 37.0 | 34.0 | 36.0 | 38.0 |
|  | 35.0 | 39.0 | 37.0 | 38.0 | 34.0 |
|  | 34.0 | 40.0 | 37.0 | 38.0 | 37.0 |
|  | 37.0 | 35.0 | 32.0 | 36.0 | 32.0 |
|  | 37.0 | 39.0 | 32.0 | 35.0 | 37.0 |
|  | 32.0 | 35.0 | 37.0 | 32.0 | 36.0 |
|  | 34.0 | 34.0 | 34.0 | 35.0 | 32.0 |
|  | 38.0 | 37.0 | 36.0 | 36.0 | 33.0 |
|  | 38.0 | 40.0 | 36.0 | 36.0 | 37.0 |
|  | 34.0 | 40.0 | 33.0 | 36.0 | 32.0 |
|  | 35.0 | 39.0 | 35.0 | 38.0 | 33.0 |
|  | 37.0 | 39.0 | 33.0 | 35.0 | 35.0 |
| **Mean** | 36.1 | 37.8 | 34.7 | 35.8 | 34.5 |
| **SD** | 1.9 | 2.0 | 2.0 | 1.8 | 2.2 |

**Table 4-6** ANOVA for pilot study

SUMMARY

| Groups | Count | Sum | Average | Variance |
|---|---|---|---|---|
| Baseline | 15 | 538 | 35.86667 | 2.838095 |
| Intervention 1 | 15 | 551 | 36.73333 | 4.495238 |
| Intervention 2 | 15 | 522 | 34.8 | 2.6 |
| Intervention 3 | 15 | 523 | 34.86667 | 4.12381 |
| Intervention 4 | 15 | 535 | 35.66667 | 2.952381 |

ANOVA

| Source of variation | SS | df | MS | F | P-value | F crit |
|---|---|---|---|---|---|---|
| Between groups | 38.05333 | 4 | 9.513333 | 2.796473 | 0.032487 | 2.502656 |
| Within groups | 238.1333 | 70 | 3.401905 | | | |
| Total | 276.1867 | 74 | | | | |

The ANOVA tested the null hypothesis that the means were not different at a 0.05 alpha level, and the p-value in the ANOVA of 0.03 allowed the team to reject the null hypothesis and verify that at least one of the interventions had an effect on patient waiting times.

Assessment of ANOVA table results may be somewhat challenging, but most health professionals have been trained to watch for a p-value less than 0.05 ($p<0.05$), so the ability to identify statistically significant results in the ANOVA table may be simplified to an extent. The ANOVA table is usually reported in the format of Table 4-6. The columns in the ANOVA table, as shown in the table, are

- **Sources of variation** = the only sources of variation for an intervention among several levels is that which occurs between each group and that which occurs within each group.
  - **Between group variation** connotes the size of the difference between the group measurements, i.e. the spread or distribution of the means between each of the groups, and is related to the effect of the intervention on the different groups.
  - **Within group variation** provides information about the degree of variation within each of the test groups, i.e. the distribution of

the values within each sample, to provide an idea of the level of uniformity of each group.

- **Sum of Squares (SS)** = each data value is subtracted from its group mean, the resulting number is squared, and then all of the squared numbers are summed to yield the sum of squares for each of the two sources of variation. Larger values of SS indicate greater variation.
- **Degrees of freedom (df)** = defined as one less than the number of observations being tested. So for Table 4-6 the df for the three groups (between groups) is $3 - 1 = 2$. The within group degrees of freedom statistic is calculated by adding the df for each group $(4 - 1)$ with that of the other groups, i.e. $(4 - 1) + (4 - 1) + (4 - 1) = 9$.
- **Mean square (MS)** = the SS divided by the df; the MS for between groups – MS(between) - indicates the amount of variation attributable to interaction between samples, while within group MS – MS(within) specifies the level of variation due to differences in the samples within each group.
- **F value** = the ratio of MS (between) to MS(within); provides the basis for determining the level of significance, or p-value.
- **P-value** = the level of alpha (incorrectly rejecting the null hypothesis) risk; at the outset of an intervention, the team determines the acceptable alpha risk, often set at 0.05, or a 5% or less risk of incorrectly inferring an effect of the intervention by erroneously rejecting the null hypothesis. The p-value associated with
- **F-crit value** = the F-value associated with the p-value that would indicate a 0.05 alpha risk. The calculated F-value must be greater than the F-crit value to reject the null hypothesis.

The concept of ANOVA can sometimes be confusing because the procedure uses the process means as the subject of computation. However, the last row of the data output (Total) contains the total sum of squares and the degrees of freedom, which defines the sample variance:

$$S^2 = \frac{SS_{total}}{df}$$

The ANOVA procedure simply provides the sources of variance, i.e. within group and between group, to split out the underlying sources for the total variation in the samples. The total variation is thus composed of the variation within the groups or samples and that between the groups or samples, each of which contributes to the total. The F-value is a ratio of the Mean Square value between groups to the Mean Square within groups, and so the larger the F-value, the greater the difference between groups, indicating a significant effect. After the F-value is calculated, the level of significance can be found in a table like that at the National Institutes of Standards and Technology (NIST) website.[1]

## Regression Analysis

Regression analysis is one of the most useful statistical tools for healthcare applications. From randomized control trials in medical research to quality improvement projects, regression analysis provides the foundation for understanding relationships and identifying important factors contributing to specific outcomes. Multiple regression is based on linear regression, or in statistical parlance, least squares analysis. Linear regression relates an outcome, usually termed the "dependent variable" (Y value in Six Sigma), to a potential causative factor, termed an "independent variable" (critical x-value in Six Sigma) by evaluating data from planned experiments or pilot tests, as well as in the normal course of process measurement for quality improvement studies. As the experiment is performed, data for both the Y- and associated x-values are collected and analyzed by a technique called least squares analysis. Luckily there are many programs that perform this rather tedious mathematical procedure and provide the various statistics that can help an improvement team understand the strength, direction, and statistical validity of the relationship between the independent and dependent variables. Multiple regression analysis performs this analysis on several independent variables at the same time, making it a powerful way of evaluating not just the effect of individual independent variables on an outcome, but also the effect of interactions of the variables on the dependent variable. For this reason, a multiple regression analysis of a process provides a wealth of data that can be used during the Analyze Phase as a way of identifying the most important critical-x values to better direct the efforts in the next phase of DMAIC—Improve. Multiple regression helps identify those critical x-values that will create the greatest change as a result of improvement initiatives.

### Simple Linear Regression

For simple linear regression, a dependent variable is compared to one associated independent variable, and the data are analyzed using the least squares technique. Simple linear regression lends itself to the use of the scatterplot (sometimes termed the scatter diagram) that plots the dependent variable (Y) with the independent variable (x) as shown in Figure 4-3. Recall that the scatterplot in Figure 4-3 was used to help define the Pearson correlation coefficient, but this plot is also useful in understanding linear regression. In fact, one of the capabilities in Microsoft Excel involves the addition of a least squares linear fit for a scatterplot, as shown in **Figure 4-8**, which is the scatterplot from Figure 4-3 with the linear regression line fitted to the plot. The equation for the line is provided on the graph:

$$Y = -0.0669x + 49.775$$

The form of this equation should be familiar from high school algebra: y = mx + b, where y is the dependent variable, m is the slope of the line, and b is the intersection with the y-axis. The following inferences can be made from the equation:

- The relationship between the dependent and independent variables is inverse (i.e., as the x-value increases, the Y-value decreases).
- The effect of the independent variable on the outcome is relatively small, since m = 0.0669. In other words, for every one unit change in x, the corresponding change in Y is only approximately 0.07.

The other reported statistic is the $R^2$ value of 0.1008. $R^2$ provides information about how well the line describes the data set, often called the "goodness

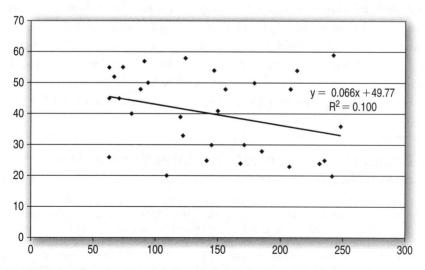

**FIGURE 4-8** Scatterplot with least squares linear regression overlay

of fit." The line represents an approximation of the data in the model, as can be seen on the scatter diagram. Since not all the scatter plot points are on the line in Figure 4-8, the line serves only as an approximation of the data, and the equation that defines the line is sometimes called a "model" of the process. The $R^2$ value indicates how well the model describes the actual underlying data, and the value typically ranges from 0 to 1. If the $R^2$ is 0, then the model does not describe the data set at all, and the $R^2$ value of 1 indicates a perfect fit (i.e., every data point falls on the line described by the equation).

**Multiple Regression**

It is fairly unusual to have a situation in which only one critical x-value is important. Most situations in healthcare organizations have multiple factors that affect a dependent variable, and it would be untenable to try to analyze each of those factors sequentially using simple linear regression. Multiple regression was designed to handle these situations, and this technique is one of the most frequently used and useful statistical procedures applied to management in the healthcare industry.

$R^2$ is also interpreted as the proportion of variation in the dependent (Y) variable explained by the independent (x) variable. As before, values will range between 0 and 1, with values closer to zero indicating little explanatory value by the x variable and values closer to 1 indicating that the x-value explains the variation in Y to a much greater degree. Thus, the $R^2$ value of 0.1008 in the linear model in Figure 4-8 indicates that about 10% of the variation in Y can be explained by changes in x. The $R^2$ value is an important factor in deciding whether to adopt a regression model, and the levels at which the model is considered useful vary by the type of model being considered. For example, a regression analysis of data from a social science study might be satisfied with an $R^2$ value of 0.4, while a controlled experiment in a laboratory setting may not be satisfied with an $R^2$ value less than 0.8.

## Example 4-5 Surgical site infections in the obstetrics unit after Caesarean section

Surgical site infections (SSIs) at Mothers and Babies Hospital have trended upward over the past two years, and the team is trying to understand the most significant factors causing the infections. The team has several months of data with each C-section associated with the physician performing the procedure, the surgical team that supported the procedure, the operating room in which the procedure was performed, and the nursing shift during which the surgery was conducted with the outcome variable (SSI) reported for each combination of factors. A multiple regression analysis was performed with the results in Table 4-7.

The team noted the highlighted data in the table (i.e., the $R^2$ value, the p-values, and the coefficients) which provided them with insight into potential causes of the increased infection rate. First, the $R^2$ value indicates that only 19% of the variation in SSIs is explained by the variables included in the analysis. The regression analysis was performed at an alpha level of 0.05, and so p-values less than 0.05 are considered significant. The only variable that has a $p < 0.05$ is Surgical Team 1, and the coefficient of +0.45 indicates that when Surgical Team 1 was involved in the procedure, the likelihood of an SSI increased substantially. The other indicators had p-values that were not statistically significant, and so the team's focus turned to Surgical Team 1 as a possible factor in the increased rate of SSIs after C-sections. The team realized, though, that the $R^2$ value of 0.19 indicates that other, unstudied factors are likely of importance, and so they also started another data review to identify those other factors.

# BRAINSTORMING IN THE ANALYZE PHASE

This technique, described in detail in Chapter 2, is used during the Analyze Phase to help generate a list of options based on the data collected in the Measure Phase. Thus, in **Example 4-5**, as the team determined that Surgical Team 1 appeared to influence SSIs unfavorably, the team may perform a brainstorming session to identify factors related to that observation. Alternatively, the team might also perform a Root Cause Analysis to hone in on the reasons for these results. Another use of brainstorming in Example 4-5 might be to start the search for other factors that may be influencing SSIs, since the $R^2$ value of 0.19 (19%) is sufficiently low to warrant further study and data collection, even while improvement efforts focus on Surgical Team 1.

# DELIVERABLES OF THE ANALYZE PHASE

At the end of the Analyze Phase, the process should be well understood quantitatively, and root causes of process performance gaps will be clearer. The metrics that are targeted for improvement will be well defined, and appropriate targets for metric performance should be established. The deliverables thus include:

- Updated process map with points of performance gaps identified
- Root cause analysis results

**Table 4-7** Regression analysis for SSIs in Mothers and Babies Hospital

**SUMMARY OUTPUT - Mother and Babies Hospital SSI analysis**

Regression statistics

| | |
|---|---|
| Multiple R | 0.440680466 |
| R square | 0.194199273 |
| Adjusted R square | 0.158385908 |
| Standard error | 0.461105516 |
| Observations | 95 |

ANOVA

| | df | SS | MS | F | Significance F |
|---|---|---|---|---|---|
| Regression | 4 | 4.611721692 | 1.152930423 | 5.422536 | 0.000587161 |
| Residual | 90 | 19.13564673 | 0.212618297 | | |
| Total | 94 | 23.74736842 | | | |

| | Coefficients | Standard error | t Stat | P-value | Lower 95% | Upper 95% | Lower 95.0% | Upper 95.0% |
|---|---|---|---|---|---|---|---|---|
| Intercept | 0.246738234 | 0.129724208 | 1.902021507 | 0.060367 | -0.01098155 | 0.50445802 | -0.010981548 | 0.50445802 |
| Dr. A | -0.170601576 | 0.095817475 | -1.78048498 | 0.078371 | -0.36095971 | 0.01975656 | -0.360959715 | 0.019756563 |
| Surg team 1 | 0.45719212 | 0.108377176 | 4.218537803 | 5.85E-05 | 0.241883037 | 0.67250339 | 0.241883037 | 0.672503388 |
| OR 1 | -0.039705166 | 0.097770459 | -0.40610596 | 0.685629 | -0.23394325 | 0.15453292 | -0.233943247 | 0.154532915 |
| Day shift | 0.033881468 | 0.096360935 | 0.351609992 | 0.725953 | -0.15755635 | 0.22531929 | -0.157556349 | 0.225319285 |

- Final performance metric definitions
- Performance metric goals for improvement (operational and financial)
- Sources of process variation

This information is critical to the development of the improvement plan during the next phase, and an effective Analyze Phase is invaluable in helping improvement teams focus on the most important factors (critical x-values) for improvement, allowing more effective allocation of strained financial and human resources.

## DISCUSSION QUESTIONS

1. What is the purpose of the Analyze Phase of DMAIC? How does an improvement team use the output of the Analyze Phase in the improvement cycle?
2. Describe the basic elements of a root cause analysis. How is it a helpful tool in the Analyze Phase?
3. Who is credited with inventing the Fishbone diagram? Describe how the diagram is helpful during the Analyze Phase.
4. What does a Pearson correlation coefficient value of –1 indicate? Is this value inherently bad?
5. Describe a scattergram. How is this graphic used during the Analyze Phase? Can a scattergram provide any quantitative data regarding cause and effect?
6. How is a hypothesis formulated for the Analyze Phase? Describe the null hypothesis. What does "reject the null hypothesis" mean?
7. When is a t-test? How is the t-test used during the Analyze Phase?
8. Why would a team need a confidence interval for data analyzed during the Analyze Phase? How is the confidence interval calculated?
9. How is ANOVA used in the Analyze Phase? What output from ANOVA can be helpful to improvement teams?
10. How is simple linear regression used in the Analyze Phase? How does the procedure add value to the improvement team's ability to identify relationships between outcomes and process metrics?

11. Describe multiple regression. How is the technique applied during the Analyze Phase? What is the difference between multiple regression and simple linear regression?
12. How does brainstorming assist the team during the Analyze Phase?

# REFERENCES

1. Upper Critical Values of the F Distribution. Accessed at http://www.itl.nist.gov/div898/handbook/eda/section3/eda3673.htm. Retrieved December 2010.

# Improve Phase Tools

## THE ESSENCE OF THE IMPROVE PHASE

In many ways, the Improve Phase is where the rubber meets the road in Six Sigma. Perhaps the biggest difference between Six Sigma and its predecessor, Plan-Do-Check-Act (PDCA), is the level of quantitative analysis and measurement performed prior to an improvement intervention; however, the Improve Phase of Six Sigma uses many of the tools in other quality frameworks like Lean and PDCA. The DMAIC approach, however, typically sets more quantitative and aggressive targets for improvement and frequently includes financial metrics in addition to operational or clinical metrics. So, for example, a project to improve the rate of surgical site infections (SSIs) will not measure just the SSI rate, but also the cost savings or revenue gains related to the rate changes. In the new environment of health care that emphasizes accountability and value-based purchasing, these financial metrics are becoming even more critical for demonstrating success of an improvement intervention. The Improve Phase focuses on designing and implementing performance enhancing initiatives, with performance measurements that subsume all relevant metrics.

## ELEMENTS OF THE IMPROVE PHASE

Since the Improve Phase uses many traditional improvement tools, it is important to understand the approaches of quality frameworks like Lean and PDCA, which include:

- Change management
- Project plan
- Failure Mode and Effects Analysis (FMEA)
- Kaizen
- 6S
- Prioritization matrix
- Deployment flowchart
- Pilot testing

Six Sigma tools offer additional resources:

- Design of experiments (DOE)
- Gauge reproducibility and repeatability (Gauge R&R described in Chapter 3)
- SIPOC impact matrix (Suppliers-Inputs-Process-Outputs-Customer, described in Chapter 2)

## FRAMEWORK FOR THE IMPROVE PHASE

The International Organization for Standardization (ISO) is a worldwide quality standards organization founded in 1947 as a consortium of national standards organizations that set international industrial and commercial standards. Its standards often become incorporated into law through treaties or national standards, and the organization has a widely used certification program that crosses many industries. Some healthcare organizations have adopted ISO as a framework for quality management. ISO standards are based on the framework shown in **Table 5-1**.

These principles can provide the context within which an Improve Phase initiative is implemented. If each one of these important issues is addressed effectively, the Improve Phase will generally be able to best determine the efficacy of a particular initiative.

**Table 5-1** ISO 9001:2008 framework for standards

| Principle | Explanation |
| --- | --- |
| Customer focus | Satisfying, or even exceeding, customer needs must be the focus of the organization. Organizations with customer focus have workers who recognize both internal and external customer requirements and devise work practices to meet customer expectations. |
| Leadership | Organizational leaders understand the mission, vision, and values, and maintain the organization's focus on those attributes. They create an internal environment to allow workers to self-actualize in ways that optimize the organization's performance. |
| Involvement of people | Engagement of the workforce has been identified as a key element of organizational performance. High functioning organizations demonstrate high levels of employee engagement. |
| Process approach | Organizations with well-defined processes improve worker understanding of their work systems and yield enhanced performance. |
| System approach to management | Processes are interrelated as a system to achieve high performance, and ultimate efficiency and effectiveness depend on optimization of the interrelated processes to maximize system output. |
| Continual improvement | Process management and improvement is a continuous effort, rather than episodic. |
| Factual approach to decision making | All decisions are based on appropriate data and analysis. |
| Mutually beneficial supplier relationships | Organizations and suppliers are interdependent and require coordination and collaboration to optimize the function of both. |

Adapted from: International Organization for Standardization. *ISO 9001:2008 Quality management principles.* Retrieved from http://www.iso.org/iso/iso_catalogue/ management_and_leadership_standards/quality_management/qmp.htm.

# TRADITIONAL IMPROVEMENT TOOLS

It is important to recognize that "traditional" does not mean "archaic." The traditional tools that are discussed in this section are not only still relevant to the Improve Phase, but in many cases essential for success.

## Change Management

To begin an initiative that creates substantive improvement, it is important to understand the challenges that come with trying to effect change. Change management is the science (and art) of managing the "people side" of change. Humans are designed for homeostasis as every clinician knows, and so changing their workflow, work environment, or work conditions will inevitably lead to resistance. Dealing with this resistance is one of the greatest challenges of the Improve Phase, so leveraging change management skills during this phase is an important key to success. Several steps in the change management process are particularly important:

- **Understand the stakeholders**–one important aspect of effecting change is understanding who will be involved in the change and how their work lives will be altered. The results of the Analyze Phase should provide insight into the departments or people involved in process change since they will be included as resources for metric operational definitions. Each of these stakeholders should become part of the solution (i.e., should be involved in the improvement project, either in planning or implementation). Additionally, the ramifications of change should be well characterized for each stakeholder or group so that they understand the impact on their jobs.
- **Identify and communicate a message about the "burning platform"**–nearly every project has a compelling underlying reason, and this rationale must be articulated well to stakeholders. A thorough understanding of this "burning platform" starts with the team, so that team members can serve as effective spokespersons throughout the organization. However, the message must not induce panic! Panic only serves to make a dysfunctional situation worse, making it even harder to create the necessary change. Thus, the burning platform message must be clear, firm, and consistent, but not shrill.
- **Articulate the proposed solution clearly**–once the burning platform message has been delivered, stakeholders will be greatly interested in

potential solutions. At that point the team should have the project proposal well developed and ready for deployment so that stakeholders can hear that there is a solution to the dilemma. A number of tools can be used to explain the proposal, such as live presentations, webinars, and sophisticated presentations like storyboards, which can be in the form of posters or as Web pages on a company intranet.

- **Update the message regularly**–not only must the project be well described and communicated initially, but progress on the improvement initiative should be communicated regularly using many of the same methods described previously. Thus, the team may have a web page on the company intranet that not only provides information to others, but there should also be a method of collecting feedback that can be used to better anticipate problems and develop proactive interventions to head off issues that could derail the project. Additionally, team members should be continually prepared to report on the project in a number of other settings, such as committee meetings and conferences that involve stakeholders. One approach to ensuring team readiness is to create a weekly "talking points" newsletter with progress updates that team members can use to update stakeholders.

- **Be prepared for resistance**–inevitably, some stakeholders will resist change. Not only is pushback expected, it also can be used constructively, so it should not necessarily be construed as negative. In some cases, some individuals will have productive feedback that can improve the project, so if resistance arises, it is best not to dismiss it as obstinance, but rather consider the issue seriously. For those issues that fall into the category of "resistance without merit," the communication strategy should have the rationale for the issue using data or the mission of the project as described in the project charter. One of the keys to overcoming the natural resistance to change is maintaining a respectful, but firm approach to those who are resisting the new order. Additionally, ensuring a consistent message based on the data that identified the need for change can reduce confusion and help those who must incorporate the changes into their work lives be better equipped to make the transition.

Change management capability is one of the most important skills that a quality professional can have, since all the analysis and measurement performed in the first three phases of DMAIC come together in the Improve Phase and require sometimes monumental change in longstanding processes.

## Project Plan

The Six Sigma team has already created a project charter for the DMAIC activity during the Define Phase described in Chapter 2. Now, the team needs to create a "mini-charter" for the improvement initiative(s) that will be undertaken during this phase. The format for the project plan is similar to that of the charter, as shown in **Table 5-2**. Since the Improve Phase may involve more than one improvement initiative, each effort should have its own project plan so that the team can track results and separate the effects of one initiative from another.

**Table 5-2** Project "mini-charter" format

| Section | Description |
|---------|-------------|
| Background and Purpose | • Brief description of the process that has led to this project recommendation<br>• Priority of the project for the Improve Phase |
| Goal statement | • Goal of this initiative (e.g., improvement of a particular metric or outcome) |
| Scope | • Work processes, departments, or personnel to be involved in the project<br>• Time period for the project<br>• Budget for the project activities |
| Team | • Core team members and consultants<br>• Supporting team members and staff |
| Improvement process | • Process steps involved in the initiative and details of the intervention, including flowchart with targeted steps highlighted<br>• Process improvement tools to be employed |
| Metrics | • Performance measures—a list of all measures that will be used to assess the project, including targets indicating successful completion |
| Support services required | • Any required services, equipment, or other resources required that have not already been mentioned |

The project plan formulates the approaches for process improvement and outlines an implementation strategy. The document rarely is more than a few pages long, but importantly it helps direct the team in implementing the process improvement. The plan serves as a guide to include the major issues encompassed in the Improve Phase:

- Confirmation of key process inputs (critical x-values) that affect the process outputs (Y) and cause defects
- Verify an acceptable range for each critical x-value to ensure that Critical To Quality (CTQ) output characteristics meet customer requirements
- Identify process adjustments (i.e., improvement initiatives, to adjust critical x variables to improve the output [Y])
- Try to predict the effects of the changes in the critical x-values and their effect on the Y value based on the relationships derived during the Analyze Phase
- Validate the measurement system (Gauge R&R)
- Implement the improvement initiative
- Validate that the effects of the changes in critical x-values had the predicted effect on Y; if not, then consider changes to the model developed during the Analyze Phase
- Verify the new process is working as expected

Each of these issues should be specifically addressed as part of the project plan, and as should be clear, much of the information comes from the Define, Measure, and Analyze work done before. Using the information, combined with the SIPOC approach described later in the chapter, the team can create a project plan that ensures robust implementation of the improvement intervention.

## Failure Mode and Effects Analysis (FMEA)

This technique, described in more detail in Chapter 3, is a helpful tool for defining each project as the plan is being developed. Recall that FMEA (sometimes called FMECA if a criticality index or Risk Priority Number is calculated) is a method of performing a "reverse Root Cause Analysis" (i.e., FMEA is used to anticipate problems and errors before any process changes are implemented). As the improvement initiatives are defined, the team can use FMEA as a way of anticipating the effect on the process, determining if errors or untoward outcomes are likely, and then redesigning the intervention to mitigate those potential failure modes. Adding this step to the Improve Phase often shortens pilot testing procedures and saves money, since failure modes are dealt with prospectively, rather than managed during implementation of the changes. The procedure is described in detail in Chapter 3.

## Kaizen

Lean and Six Sigma are highly complementary, and the application of Kaizen to the Improve Phase is a good example of this synergy. The use of Kaizen started in Japan, and the approach is used as a way of achieving ongoing, continuous improvement. Rather than trying to generate innovative, revolutionary change, Kaizen focuses on creating for rapid incremental change. A "Kaizen event" allocates time to a rapid cycle improvement team to focus on a specific intervention or group of interventions. The Kaizen event focuses on creating the project plan and executing it within a week, so the scope of the project must be sized appropriately to allow completion of the intervention within the one-week time period. As implementation proceeds, the team tracks metrics to determine the need to make rapid corrections to the Kaizen plan.

Kaizen events rely on basic management principles for success:

- **Worker empowerment**–team members and workers involved in the event must feel empowered to "tweak" the process and provide feedback to the team on which interventions are effective and which are not. For example, if a process improvement has produced spectacular results on outcomes but at a cost of worker satisfaction, the affected workers need to feel that they can bring issues to the team for consideration, rather than find that their issues are ignored.
- **Just in time learning**–workers often must learn new skills to make an intervention successful, such as using data to track performance, and the training for these skills needs to be close to the time and place where the skills will be applied. The Kaizen event thus includes the training required for the intervention.
- **Rapid cycle improvement**–a Kaizen event is designed to facilitate planning, intervention, and measurement within one week, and so the cycle for improvement must have communication and change implementation processes that create the environment for rapid response times and the ability to change an intervention within a very short time-

frame. Completion of the project in such a short time can help improvement teams feel a sense of accomplishment that is often not as intense in longer term projects. Many teams set short-term goals (gates) to determine if the event will meet the timeline and goals initially set for the improvement, and if a particular short term goal is not met, then the "gate" may close and another approach implemented to avoid wasted time and resources. The team may alternatively decide that the goal was unrealistic and revise the Kaizen event plan, but in either event, the gate is not passed if the project fails to meet the short-term goal.

- **Jidoka (autonomation)**–a uniquely Japanese concept, Jidoka describes the use of machines to detect defects and stop the process before the defect is propagated through to a patient. For example, inline monitors for $CO_2$ in a ventilator tubing connection detect rising $CO_2$ levels in the patient's exhalations and alert caregivers of the need to change ventilator settings. Numerous examples like this exist in health care, and increasingly automation has been a major factor in the effort to improve patient safety. Kaizen events target opportunities such as these to leverage and implement automation tools to improve processes for patient care.

## Conducting a Kaizen Event

These events require preparation to be successful, and the team may spend substantial time addressing several issues prior to the actual event:

- **Focus**–a Kaizen event during the Improve Phase will focus on a specific improvement intervention that can be achieved within one week. Information from the Define, Measure, and Analyze Phases will likely be well understood by this time, but a summary of the data that created the priorities for change should be readily available so that the team maintains focus on the improvement initiative and not debate nuances in the data.
- **Priorities and scope**–the team will have priorities set from the previous phases, but the Kaizen event should reiterate and reinforce the mandates for change so that improvement teams understand that they have organizational support for their efforts. Just as important, though, is the need to set the scope of the project to avoid reaching too far and discovering later that the project is unachievable. The improvement activities must be directed at the interventions that are most likely to

have the greatest positive impact on the customer (i.e., improved safety, reduced costs, faster throughput and response time, and reduction of defects). The flowchart and prioritization matrix can help establish these focal points, and in some cases use of a value stream map, which is a specialized type of flowchart that provides additional insight into process flow. On the other hand, setting project scope is also a key element of planning a Kaizen event. Holding fast to a one-week timeline for completion of the project will set boundaries and avoid the natural tendency to add "just one more thing" to the scope of the event.

- **Team selection**–the appropriate team is crucial to the Kaizen event's success, starting with the size of the team. The team should be of sufficient size to accomplish all of the goals of the Kaizen, but not so large as to be unmanageable. Representation from multiple departments and disciplines is often needed, and it is usually safer to over-represent in the early stages of planning, rather than miss an important participant in the process. The same principles for team selection and structure that were described in Chapter 2 apply to team selection for a Kaizen event. Importantly, team membership must include at least one or more people from the target process on the Kaizen team, both as a reality check for proposed changes and for ensuring continuity of the new process once the Kaizen event has concluded.

- **Training**–nearly all Kaizen events will require new skills or process knowledge, and training is a key characteristic of a successful program. In some cases, the entire first day of the event is spent in training sessions to prepare the team for the rest of the week. Training sessions may include specific procedures that are changing as part of the process improvement, or they might center on quality improvement techniques that will be applied as part of the interventions.

- **Tracking**–every project requires tracking to determine if goals are being met, and use of an Excel® spreadsheet with goals, metrics, and an indication of whether the project is on schedule. An example spreadsheet is shown in **Figure 5-1**, and a working copy of the spreadsheet can be downloaded from the publisher's website. The spreadsheet contains macros that require at least Excel 2007 or newer.

The Kaizen team's activities must be highly orchestrated to ensure meeting the timeline and target performance. The agenda of the workshop is outlined in **Table 5-3**.

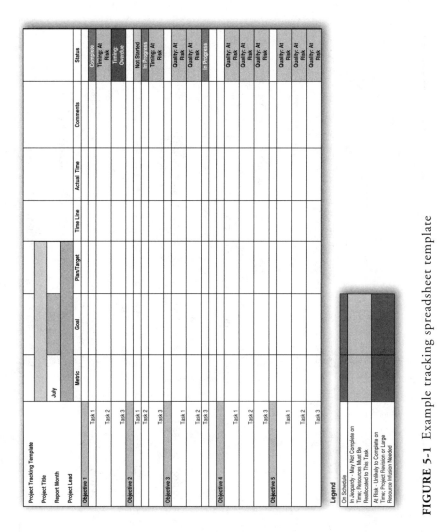

**FIGURE 5-1** Example tracking spreadsheet template

Notably, senior managers must sponsor the event and participate both during and at the end of the week. Not only does this involvement provide senior leaders with insight into operations and staff, but it also demonstrates management commitment to improvement and allows managers to engage workers in a positive way for significant improvement. Kaizen leaders should encourage team members to make as many of the presentations as possible to demonstrate staff capabilities and also to acquaint senior managers with line staff. Team engagement is empowering for staffers who may not have much interaction with senior leaders.

**Table 5-3** Kaizen event agenda

| Day | Time | Task | Comment |
| --- | --- | --- | --- |
| 1 | 8:00 - 8:15 | Introductions and overview of project | Presentation of DMA phase information sheets, introduction of team |
| | 8:15 - 9:00 | Ground rules and spirit of improvement | Expectations for team, including rules of engagement (e.g., stay on topic, no personal attacks, etc.) |
| | 9:00 -12:00 | Classroom training | Specific training regarding skills needed in improvement effort |
| | 12:00 -1:00 | Lunch | |
| | 1:00 - 3:00 | Classroom training | Specific training regarding skills needed in improvement effort |
| | 4:00 – 4:45 | Process walk-through | Walk through process to be improved to identify targets for improvement through VSM diagram or PERT chart |
| | 4:45 - 5:00 | Debrief | Review day's progress, allow people to vent regarding the process, reports on findings |
| 2 | 8:15 - 10:00 | Complete current state process map | VSM or PERT chart completed by team through group effort to identify current process with workarounds, defects in process steps |
| | 10:00 - 12:00 | Discuss / develop future state process map | Identify targets for intervention, develop ideal process map with associated metrics, interventions for improvements, team member assignments, timeline for implementation |
| | 12:00 - 1:00 | Working lunch: Present future vision and goals to management | Working lunch with senior management sponsors to discuss interventions and goals |
| | 1:00 - 4:45 | Begin implementation | Organize teams, develop task lists, populate scorecards for implementation |
| | 4:45 - 5:00 | Debrief | Review day's progress, barriers, and successes |

**Table 5-3** Kaizen event agenda (*continued*)

| Day | Time | Task | Comment |
|---|---|---|---|
| 3 | 8:00 - 8:15 | Review and develop day's action plan | Review each team's scorecard, develop altered plans if required, outline day's tasks |
| 4 | 8:15 - 4:45 | Continue implementation | Team implementation of interventions |
|   | 4:45 - 5:00 | Debrief | Review day's progress, barriers, and successes |
|   | 8:00 - 8:15 | Review and develop day's action plan | Review each team's scorecard, develop altered plans if required, outline day's tasks |
|   | 8:15 - 4:45 | Continue implementation | Team implementation of interventions |
|   | 4:45 - 5:00 | Debrief | Review day's progress, barriers, and successes |
| 5 | 8:00 - 8:15 | Review and develop day's action plan | Review each team's scorecard, develop altered plans if required, outline day's tasks |
|   | 8:15 - 11:00 | Complete implementation | Team implementation of interventions |
|   | 12:00 - 1:00 | Working lunch: Develop report and long-term action items | Each intervention group organizes reports for management and identifies remaining issues for further improvement |
|   | 1:00 - 2:00 | Report of accomplishments to management, including process walk | Reports to senior management sponsors, may include a process walk through |
|   | 2:00 - 4:30 | Complete final details | Final recommendations and report created |
|   | 4:30 - 5:00 | Celebrate accomplishments and adjourn | Finalize project |

## 6S

5S is a tool to better organize the workplace to make improvements more easily implemented. However, the technique is also used to avoid waste. 5S is the original term originally used by Hiroyuki Hirano as part of the Toyota Production System,[1] but as health care has adopted the approach, it has become 6S, signifying:

- **Sort**–determine what is needed to accomplish work and what is not needed; remove the unneeded items
- **Straighten**–find a place for all needed items and ensure that everything is put in its place
- **Shine**–clean the workplace and keep it clean
- **Standardize**–develop a system to apply the first three S's to the entire workplace
- **Sustain**–develop processes to maintain the gains, i.e. to ensure that the workplace stays in order
- **Safety**–eliminate hazards and dangerous workplace features

6S is a tool not just directed at organizing and maintaining an orderly workplace, but it is also useful for building teams within a common work area. Additionally, it reduces the time wasted looking for needed items to complete a task (e.g., the annoying search for a patient's chart or lab results in an office) and eliminates the frustrations that accompany these fruitless searches. Just as with Kaizen events that target specific parts of a process to improve quickly, 6S events get everyone in a work area focused on a specific task of reducing clutter and organizing the workspace to make the environment more pleasant and the work easier to complete. 6S event teams can realize a tangible sense of accomplishment as they view the new work environment, and that feeling often translates into greater team cohesion and productivity. Simply cleaning a workplace is not the only goal of 6S–the technique requires an understanding of the workflow that will occur in the workspace so that as items go through the Straighten step they can be laid out to facilitate flow in the space. Another important feature of 6S is to label everything in the workspace with understandable stickers or markers to expedite finding items or quickly recognizing items that are out of place. Example 5-1 describes the use of 6S in a lab environment.

## Example 5-1 6S in a lab setting

The lab team at the Shipshape Pediatric Clinic faced another round of cost cutting. As the team grappled with the lower budget figures, they looked around the lab and were rather astounded at how cluttered it had become. Each time a new lab test was introduced into the mix, the team found an open spot in the lab and plunked the test instruments and materials into that spot. The resulting disorganization was remarkable. Out of curiosity, the team rummaged through the disposable supplies, particularly those that had expiration dates, and they found that a little over a third of the supplies had passed their expiration date because they had been covered by newer supplies in a drawer where disposables were kept. The team then looked at the typical groups of tests that they performed on patients in the clinics and then reviewed the positions of the equipment in the lab. It surprised them that the equipment was arranged in a way that increased the movement of the lab specimens, extended the time needed to perform analyses, and decreased throughput. That was enough for the team leader. The estimate was nearly $20,000 in expired supplies, reduced productivity compared to benchmarks, and diminished physician and patient satisfaction due to waiting times for tests. The team leader organized a 6S event that directed the team to think first about the workflow in the lab, and then how to arrange the lab to optimize flow through the lab. They began with a Sort step, which identified all the "detritus" that had built up in the lab over several years, red-tagged the items, and removed them to another area for disposition. The Straighten step was even more productive. The team evaluated what lab tests were done in order of frequency and rearranged the lab equipment to create a stepwise flow of the specimens through the lab. Placing the appropriate disposable items next to each workstation was another favorable change, and then arranging the disposables in the drawers so that older items were in the front of the drawer so that they were selected first virtually eliminated the problem of expired dates. After a thorough cleaning (Shine step), the team leader established a checklist for daily inspection of the lab to ensure that items stayed in their proper locations (Standardize), and an inventory management system to flag disposable items that seem to be ordered too frequently (Sustain). Additionally, the team established metrics to monitor lab accident rates (Safety).

### Conducting a 6S Event

As with a Kaizen event, preparation makes a big difference in the success of the 6S event. The goals are similar—to achieve improvements in a work system—but the approach in a 6S event is much more focused on the six issues within the 6S construct. Where a Kaizen event takes a more holistic quality improvement approach, the 6S event concentrates on the work environment and the six issues in 6S. The phases of a 6S event are listed in **Table 5-4**.

During the planning phase, the project leader determines the issues to be addressed in the event and assembles a team to begin work on solutions. Issues may be discovered in a number of ways (e.g., by request from

**Table 5-4**  6S event phases

| Phase | Tasks | Timeline |
|---|---|---|
| Planning | Identify problem | |
| | Select team | |
| | Collect data<br>- Photos of workspace<br>- Quantifiable costs associated with workspace disorder | 1 hour |
| | Set targets and scope | 1 hour |
| Implementation | Conduct training<br>- 6S tools and concepts<br>- Concepts of waste<br>- 6S improvement process<br>- Metrics | 1.5 hours |
| | Team walk through to observe workspace<br>- Look for waste<br>- Look for safety issues<br>- Completion of 6S evaluation form (Figure 5-2) | 1 hour |
| | Consolidate team observations | 0.5 hour |
| | Team meeting to address targets | 1 hour |
| | Apply intervention | 4 hours |
| Post-implementation | Post-intervention walk through<br>- Collect metrics and compare with pre-intervention<br>- Photos of workspace<br>- Completion of 6S evaluation forms | 0.5 hour |
| | Develop plan to sustain | 1.5 hours |

a manager, through productivity data for a specific work unit, or from safety reports indicating increased risk in a particular area). Team selection should reflect the nature of the problem, but the team should always include workers from the area of interest and then appropriate members from other departments to address specific issues (e.g., patient safety). The project leader can usually do the initial data collection for a 6S project, which includes photos of the workspace and any data that indicates the effect of the current lack of order on cost or revenue, throughput, or other parameters such as customer satisfaction. Once the data are collected, the project manager can work with other managers to establish goals for particular metrics, based either on industry benchmarks or on company objectives set by senior management.

The implementation phase of a 6S event calls upon specific tools designed for this process, as shown in **Table 5-5**. A blank 6S evaluation form is provided as **Figure 5-2**. These approaches leverage team experience and a good understanding of process workflow to accomplish 6S goals. Example 5-1 demonstrates the application of several of these approaches.

After the event has concluded, the project manager's monitoring system will track relevant measures for a period of time determined by senior managers and team members, with an intervention plan for any lapses in performance.

**Table 5-5** 6S event tools

| 6S improvement tool | Phase | Description |
|---|---|---|
| **Red tag system** | Sort | • Red tag (or some other indicator) used by team to indicate nonessential items<br>• Red-tagged items placed in a location where other departments can determine potential usefulness<br>• After prescribed time (e.g., 1 week), red tagged items are discarded or sold |
| **Color codes** | Sort<br>Straighten | • Colors are assigned to specific classes of items<br>• Color tags or markers are placed on items during Sort phase<br>• Items are stored in appropriate place during Straighten phase |
| **Visual work instructions** | Shine<br>Standardize<br>Sustain | • Symbolic representations of workflow<br>• Succinct descriptions of steps and standards<br>• Symbolic representation of "do not" policies |
| **Workplace layout** | Shine<br>Standardize | • Review of workplace layout and rearrangement to accommodate workflow<br>• Reclamation of unused/misused space |
| **Ergonomic hazard analysis** | Straighten<br>Shine<br>Standardize | • Determine if workplace items have associated risks of injury to workers or customers<br>• Redesign or replacement of dangerous items<br>• Addition of safety materials (information and devices) to reduce hazards |
| Alternative storage analysis | Straighten<br>Shine<br>Standardize | • Analyze workspace items to determine immediacy of use<br>• Remove infrequently used items to another place (e.g., storage space) |

| Workspace: | \<Name or Description of Workspace\> | Item Score (1 – 5) | |
|---|---|---|---|
| | | Pre intervention | Post intervention |
| **Sort: Needed vs. Unneeded** | Have All Unneeded Items Been Removed? | | |
| | Are Walkways, Work Areas, Locations Identified And Marked? | | |
| | Is There A Procedure in Place for Removing Unneeded Items? | | |
| | | | |
| **Straighten: Everything in Its Place** | Is There A Place For Every Item? | | |
| | Has Every Item Been Put in Its Designated Place? | | |
| | Are Item Locations Well Marked and Identifiable? | | |
| | | | |
| **Shine: Cleaning** | Are All Workspaces Free Of Clutter and Debris? | | |
| | Are Cleaning Materials Available and Accessible? | | |
| | Are All Markers and Indicators Clean and Functional? | | |
| | Are Cleaning Schedules Posted for All Areas? | | |
| | | | |
| **Standardize: Application of 6s to Entire Workspace** | Is All Necessary Information for Proper Operations Visible and Accessible? | | |
| | Are All Standards Known and/or Posted? | | |
| | Are All Visual Displays Current? | | |
| | Are Standards Being Followed? | | |
| | | | |
| **Sustain: Processes to Maintain Gains** | Processes Well Defined and Procedures Being Followed? | | |
| | Audit And Feedback System in Place? | | |
| | Feedback Response System in Place? | | |
| | | | |
| **Safety: Incident Monitoring and Response** | Safety Monitoring Program in Place? | | |
| | Safety Equipment Accessible and Well Marked? | | |
| | Safety Risk Intervention in Place? | | |
| | | | |
| | Total Score: | | |
| Team Member: | | Date: | |

**FIGURE 5-2**  6S Evaluation Form

## Prioritization Matrix

The prioritization matrix is discussed in detail in Chapter 3, and the use of this tool extends to the Improve Phase as well. The prioritization matrix is typically used to rank several improvement interventions on the basis of how likely each is to improve the target process. The DMAIC may have several possible interventions to try during the Improve Phase, but limited resources for implementation. Sometimes priorities are clear, but if not, the prioritization matrix can help, as shown in Example 5-2.

---

# Example 5-2 Prioritization of interventions using a prioritization matrix

Bob Sechsten, a Six Sigma Black Belt (SSBB) at the HighQual Doctor's Clinic, was in the Improve Phase of a DMAIC project on improving medication dosage accuracy for drugs administered at the clinic. Because of recent data that identified pediatric drug dosing in outpatient settings as a significant patient safety risk, Bob was tasked with measuring the sigma level of the pediatric dosing process, and his data indicated a performance level of $3.5\sigma$. The clinic's physicians were not satisfied with this rate, and so Bob was asked to evaluate the dose calculation and medication administration process and find interventions to lower the error rate. Bob assembled a team that evaluated the process and developed four potential interventions, but the team was unable to prioritize the interventions, since there were multiple parameters to consider – cost, expected impact, staff capability, training requirements, disruption of workflow, and time for completion. He developed a prioritization matrix (shown in **Figure 5-3**) that accounted for each of these parameters and assigned weights according to their relative importance and impact on the decision. So, for example, the cost parameter has a weight of $-0.5$ because it is inversely related to rank and of intermediate importance to the project leaders and sponsors. From the priority matrix, the team determined that Intervention 4 would be the first implemented.

---

The prioritization matrix can serve a useful function during the Improve Phase, helping the team to better focus implementation decisions.

## Deployment Flowchart

The process for creating a deployment flowchart was described in Chapter 3, and this flowchart is highly useful during the implementation of initiatives during the Improve Phase. Recall that the purpose of the deployment flowchart is to clarify accountability for specific steps in a process. To ensure that each initiative is carried out decisively, participants in the project need to understand their specific tasks and accountabilities. Additionally, the

HighQual Clinic Medication Error Reduction Project

| | Parameter | Cost (in Thousands) | Impact | Staff Capability | Training Requirements | Workflow Disruption | Completion Time (Days) | Weighted Score | Rank |
|---|---|---|---|---|---|---|---|---|---|
| | Weight | −0.5 | 1 | 0.75 | −0.5 | −0.4 | −0.3 | | |
| **Intervention** | | | | | | | | | |
| 1 | Raw | 5 | 6 | 4 | 3 | 4 | 90 | | |
| | Weighted | −2.5 | 6 | 3 | −1.5 | −1.6 | −27 | −23.6 | 3 |
| 2 | Raw | 3 | 3 | 5 | 5 | 7 | 120 | | |
| | Weighted | −1.5 | 3 | 3.75 | −2.5 | −2.8 | −36 | −36.05 | 4 |
| 3 | Raw | 12.5 | 8 | 7 | 7 | 3 | 42 | | |
| | Weighted | −6.25 | 8 | 5.25 | −3.5 | −1.2 | −12.6 | −10.3 | 2 |
| 4 | Raw | 1.1 | 3 | 8 | 2 | 5 | 12 | | |
| | Weighted | −0.55 | 3 | 6 | −1 | −2 | −3.6 | 1.85 | 1 |

(Score)

**FIGURE 5-3** Prioritization matrix for HighQual Clinic

deployment flowchart is a very useful way to inform process owners and users of their new responsibilities in the transformed process, as shown in Example 5-3.

Deployment flowcharts have the potential of clarifying roles in an improved process and comprise an important tool for the Improve Phase.

---

### Example 5-3 Deployment flowcharts in the Improve Phase

The Kaizen team at the Six Saints Hospital has been directed to focus on the emergency department (ED) triage process, and they have found several points of duplicated effort in the process of getting the patient to an exam room to see the doctor, as shown in a high level flowchart in **Figure 5-4**.

The team created the deployment flowchart shown in **Figure 5-5**, which effectively demonstrated which staff members performed the steps in the current process. Working with the staff, the team identified extra steps that slowed patient throughput and did not add value.

The revised workflow removed one of the nursing evaluations (the step before prior authorization is obtained) and completed all of the administrative steps before clinical involvement as shown in **Figure 5-6**. The staff duties are clearly defined in the deployment flowchart, making it easy for the ED staff to understand the new sequence of events.

---

## Pilot Testing

Before major changes in a process are deployed, many teams utilize pilot testing to understand unanticipated consequences of changes in the process on other steps or processes in the organization. Pilot testing involves a trial run of changes in a process on a smaller subset of the population affected by the process. For instance, the improvements made to the ED admission process in Example 5-3 may be tried on one shift for a week to determine if the approach caused any problems with waiting times or effectiveness of the triage process. Many pilot tests are conducted during a less busy time to avoid disruption from the changed process. During the pilot test, the improvements can be fine-tuned to ameliorate any problems that arise, as well as collect data to demonstrate that the changes in the process have the anticipated effects. Feedback from process owners and users during the pilot test is crucial for determining if the improvements are effective or if they cause abrasion with staff or customers.

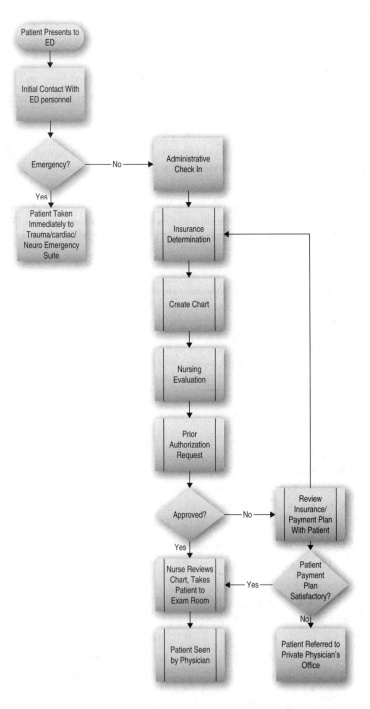

**FIGURE 5-4** Flowchart of Registration Process (Example 5-3)

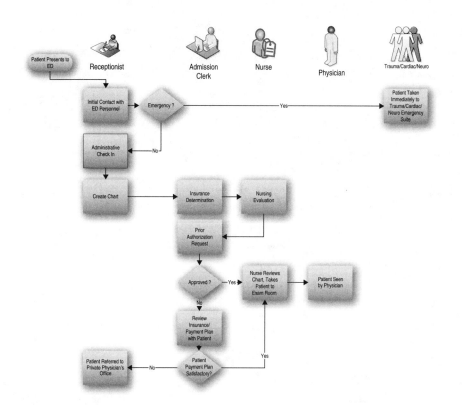

**FIGURE 5-5** Deployment flowchart for current ED admission process

A critical component of a pilot test is the selection of metrics to track and targets for improvement appropriate for the sample size in the pilot. Metrics may include:

- **Process measures** like throughput, staffing ratios, productivity statistics, wait times, turnaround times
- **Outcome measures** like clinical services used, costs, patient clinical status, clinical benchmark measures (e.g., those required by the Centers for Medicare and Medicaid Services), compliance metrics (e.g., meeting certain thresholds for critical measures like pressure ulcers or surgical site infections)
- **Satisfaction metrics** like patient and staff satisfaction survey results

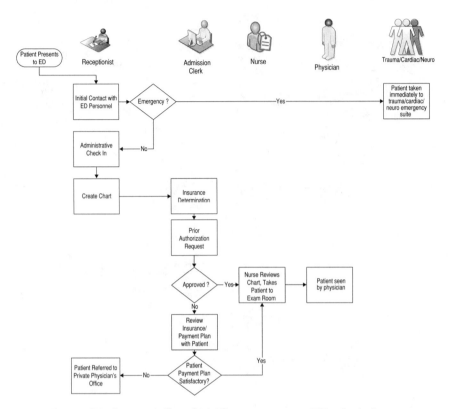

**FIGURE 5-6** Deployment flowchart for new process ED admission

Pilot testing is a common approach across many industries from software development to soap manufacturing, and the use of the procedure to reduce costs and ensure safety of a new process or a significant improvement in an existing process makes it a compelling method for the Improve Phase. The lessons learned during the pilot test are directly applied to the implementation plan is one of the important deliverables from the Improve Phase.

## Six Sigma Tools

When Six Sigma was formulated by Bill Smith of Motorola in 1986, the goal was to improve productivity by reducing errors to nearly zero. The "traditional" improvement tools discussed in the prior section were available to him and were incorporated into the DMAIC concept, but to achieve Six Sigma levels of performance, higher levels of precision and accuracy were needed, necessitating the use of more advanced approaches, such as:

- Design of Experiments (DOE)
- Gauge reproducibility and repeatability (Gauge R&R)
- SIPOC impact matrix

These approaches have evolved as the Six Sigma paradigm has matured, and their use in performance improvement has advanced the science of quality, as well as increasing focus on customers.

## Design of Experiments

An experiment is a systematic procedure carried out under controlled conditions to uncover an unknown effect or to test a hypothesis (such as the null hypothesis discussed in Chapter 4). Although not a technique specifically developed for Six Sigma, DOE has been most extensively applied in Six Sigma projects to ensure that the analyses performed meet a requisite level of statistical rigor. The DOE process uses the information gathered and analyzed during the Define, Measure, and Analyze phases to develop an approach to evaluating possible improvements in a process. DOE resonates with many healthcare managers who have scientific backgrounds and who understand the scientific method. Although the gold standard for experiments in medical research is the randomized control trial (RCT) in which a single variable is changed while all others are held constant, the application of the scientific method in quality improvement rarely lends itself to that level of control because of the time and expense required to perform an RCT. Additionally, in complex processes or systems, the interaction of independent variables (critical x's) may influence the outcome variable (Y) as much as any individual variable alone. Statistical methods have been developed that allow several variables and their interactions to be tested simultaneously with a level of confidence like that obtained with RCTs.

Designed experiments in the Improve Phase specifically seek to determine which critical x values, or factors, have a significant impact on the Y value, or response variable, in the fundamental Six Sigma equation described in Chapter 3. Factors are those critical x-values that are controllable in an experiment, and varying the factors in the experiment can determine what levels of each critical x are necessary to optimize the output. These optimal levels of each of the critical x-values are then applied in the final implementation plan for the process. The designed experiment may be performed prior to a pilot test or can actually comprise the pilot test.

---

## Example 5-4 DOE during the Improve Phase

The pediatric clinical improvement team had finished the Define, Measure, and Analyze phases of their Six Sigma project to eliminate dosage errors in children in the hospital's outpatient department. The team identified three key critical x-values that lead to errors and defined two potential interventions for each of the three critical x-values (factors) as shown in **Figure 5-7**. There are two levels for the three interventions, which is called a $2^3$ (pronounced "two by three") factorial experiment, because there are three factors, each of which has two levels. The table in the figure shows every combination of levels (designated as −1 and +1) of the three factors and requires eight trials. The team was able to perform the eight trials and determined the significance of each factor and level, and that information was used to revise the process. The optimal combination of factors and levels was then pilot tested in the pediatric oncology clinic, finalized, and then deployed throughout the entire outpatient department.

---

Example 5-4 illustrates how the use of DOE in the Improve Phase allows the evaluation of several critical x-values simultaneously, providing information not just about each factor individually, but also about combinations of factors that can cause interaction effects. The $2^3$ design is commonly used, since addition of factors and levels increases the number of trials necessary for evaluation of the factors exponentially. If larger numbers of factors and/or levels are needed, an approach known as fractional factorial design is

| Trial Number | Critical x-values | | |
|:---:|:---:|:---:|:---:|
| | Factor 1 | Factor 2 | Factor 3 |
| 1 | −1 | −1 | −1 |
| 2 | +1 | −1 | −1 |
| 3 | −1 | +1 | −1 |
| 4 | +1 | +1 | −1 |
| 5 | −1 | −1 | +1 |
| 6 | +1 | −1 | +1 |
| 7 | −1 | +1 | +1 |
| 8 | +1 | +1 | +1 |

**FIGURE 5-7** DOE Example–Medication Dosage Error Prevention

employed to reduce the number of trials needed to gain the needed information. A more detailed discussion of DOE can be found in the *Advanced Performance Improvement in Health Care* text by Lighter.[2]

## Gauge R&R

As measurements are being made in the Improve Phase to determine the effects of an improvement needs to be statistically significant, which means that the methods and instruments of measurement must be well calibrated for precise and accurate measurement. Gauge R&R, discussed in depth in Chapter 3, measures the level of variation in measurements due to the imprecision of the measurement system, using statistical techniques like analysis of variance (ANOVA, described in Chapter 4), and then compares this "measurement system variation" to the total observed variation to determine the precision and accuracy of the measurement system. When performing measurements at the Six Sigma (3 ppm) level, even tiny errors introduced by the measurement system can skew results and lead to incorrect inferences. Thus, gauge R&R is an important component of the Improve Phase of a Six Sigma project.

## SIPOC Impact Matrix

SIPOC, described in Chapter 2, is a useful tool in the Improve Phase for understanding the effects of an improvement initiative on each component of the value chain. Although improvement projects usually focus on the P, or Process, portion of SIPOC, the upstream and downstream effects of the project may be significant and should be considered as part of the project plan. Thus, a SIPOC impact matrix can help the team think through the entire value stream to anticipate and avoid potentially detrimental effects.

---

# Example 5-5 Use of SIPOC impact matrix in an Improve Phase intervention

The Kaizen team at Six Saints Hospital (Example 5-3) is ready to pilot their interventions after a rigorous planning period, and as one of the final steps prior to the pilot, they created a SIPOC impact matrix to anticipate effects on the value chain. The matrix in **Figure 5-8** demonstrates some of the effects anticipated for each of the stakeholders and elements of the SIPOC chain.

| Suppliers | | | |
|---|---|---|---|
| Referring Physicians | **Ambulance Companies** | | |
| Pre-screening via Telephone | No Expected Impact | | |

| Inputs | | | |
|---|---|---|---|
| Referrals | **Patients** | | |
| Referrals Encouraged Through Pre-screening | Rapid Intervention and Classification | | |

| Process | | | |
|---|---|---|---|
| Receptionist | **Admission Clerk** | **Nurse** | **Physician** |
| Expectation of Rapid Throughput to Triage System | Training to Recognize Urgency of Patient Condition to Ensure Rapid Processing | More Rapid Throughput Required Due to Upstream Efficiencies | Should Improve Patient Availability and Decrease Physician Downtime |

| Output | |
|---|---|
| Patient | **Private Physician** |
| Increased Patient Satisfaction Due to More Rapid Processing Possible Patient Abrasion Due to Feeling "Rushed" | Improved Reporting for Follow Up Patient Records Available Within 24 Hours Improved Referring and Follow Up Physician Satisfaction |

| Customer | |
|---|---|
| Patient | **Payer** |
| Improved Satisfaction Improved Loyalty Improved Willingness to Recommend | Possible Abrasion Regarding Higher Volumes Improved Member Satisfaction with Provider May Enhance Payer's Image |

**FIGURE 5-8** SIPOC Impact Matrix

The SIPOC impact matrix focuses the improvement team on unanticipated consequences for all of the people and systems in the value chain, and is a valuable tool as one of the final steps prior to implementing an improvement initiative.

# COMPLETING THE IMPROVE PHASE

At the end of the Improve Phase, the team has developed and tested improvement initiatives, determined the effect of the initiatives on key performance indicators, and prepared for the next step, the Control Phase. The deliverables for the Improve Phase include:

- Optimized process map
- Report of improvement initiatives
- Key performance indicators and expected system wide effects
- Prioritization of improvements for system wide deployment (if applicable)
- Implementation plan for system wide deployment
  - Risk management plan
  - Budget for deployment
  - Contingency plan for issues that may be occur during deployment

Once these deliverables are completed, the team can embark on the Control Phase.

# DISCUSSION QUESTIONS

1. What is the ISO and how are its standards relevant to the Improve Phase of DMAIC?
2. Describe the basic steps of change management and give an example of each from your experience.
3. What is a project plan? How does it differ from a project charter?
4. How is FMEA applied in the Improve Phase? Is a criticality score useful in the Improve Phase?
5. Describe a Kaizen event. How does the event help staff during the Improve Phase?
6. What is Jidoka? How has Jidoka been applied in health care?
7. Describe Just in Time Learning. How is this approach applicable in a Kaizen event?
8. What are the important elements of team selection for a Kaizen event?
9. What are the 6Ss of health care? How can 6S improve work system performance?

10. Describe a 6S event. How can a 6S team sustain the gains from the event?
11. Describe how a prioritization matrix is used in the Improve Phase.
12. Create a deployment flowchart similar to the one in Figures 5-4 and 5-5 for a process that you use every day in your work.
13. What are the advantages of pilot testing in the Improve Phase? What are the disadvantages?
14. Describe design of experiments. Why is it a crucial approach for the Improve Phase?
15. How does Gauge R&R apply to the Improve Phase?
16. What is a SIPOC impact matrix? How is it used in the Improve Phase?
17. What are the deliverables of the Improve Phase?

# REFERENCES

1. Hirano, H. (1990). *Five pillars of the visual workplace.* Portland, OR: Productivity Press.
2. Lighter, D. (2010) *Advanced performance improvement in health care: Principles and methods.* Sudbury, MA: Jones & Bartlett Learning.

# 6

# Control Phase Tools

*"A system must be managed. It will not manage itself."*

—W. Edwards Deming

*"Dr. Deming enjoys showing an advertisement for some computer software. The advertisement's headline is: 'Get in Control for Only $59.95.' He remarks: 'I think it'll take a little more than that!'"*

—Henry R. Neave

*"That which we persist in doing becomes easier, not that the task itself has become easier, but that our ability to perform it has improved."*

—Ralph Waldo Emerson

## THE ESSENCE OF THE CONTROL PHASE

A tremendous amount of work goes into the Define, Measure, Analyze, and Improve phases, and the typical Six Sigma project nets a substantial gain. Maintaining this gain and, indeed, expanding on the success is the goal of the Control Phase. At this stage of DMAIC, the team and senior leadership sponsors are primarily focused on ensuring that the improved process does not deteriorate into its prior form, or worse. Putting the revamped process in place may fix the problem in the short term, but the Control Phase deploys approaches that monitor the process effectively and

**175**

reacts quickly to signs of impending deterioration. Additionally, the tools of the Control Phase may even suggest opportunities for further improvement as the environment changes.

## ELEMENTS OF THE CONTROL PHASE

The Control Phase is dedicated to ensuring that the improvements that were tested and proven during the Improve Phase are institutionalized and sustained. Improvement projects that end with substantive gains are successes to be sustained, and the Control Phase tools are designed to set up the monitoring and continuous improvement processes to ensure that these gains are not only maintained, but also enhanced as new opportunities for improvement become apparent. Most of the tools have been discussed in previous chapters, but their application in the Control Phase has different implications. The tools relevant to the Control Phase include:

- Flow charts
- Standardization and institutionalization of process changes
- Training plans and programs
- Monitoring plans
  - Poka yoke
  - Audit plans
- Control charts
- Process sigma level

The primary activities during this phase involve development of an operational plan that can be used as a roadmap for deployment of the improved process, as well as monitoring the new process to ensure that the gains made by the improvement are not lost as the new process is implemented throughout the enterprise.

## FRAMEWORK FOR THE CONTROL PHASE

Every organization has barriers to improvement, and the Control Phase must design countermeasures to deal with these obstacles before they arise. The Improve Phase applies quality improvement techniques, while the Control Phase calls upon tactics that have been developed for quality assurance. This approach, continuous quality improvement (CQI), has been honed over the years to not only ensure that any gains realized from the improvement are maintained, but also that new opportunities are recognized and exploited. In other words, the improvement process is incorporated into the quality maintenance program. Astute managers must be continually finding new opportunities for improvement while ensuring that gains in quality levels are maintained if the organization's performance is to strengthen over time. Achieving this ambitious goal requires a culture of improvement. Six Sigma helps set aggressive goals for performance (3 DPMO), and achievement of this level of performance is iterative (i.e., it is attained in steps rather than in one giant leap).

CQI has grown into an organizational philosophy that has sustained the highest performing organizations throughout the world. No longer is short-term correction of a quality lapse a solution to long-term performance. Instead, high performers now incorporate monitoring systems and improvement cycles into all products and services, and this approach spans virtually all industries, including health care. The Control Phase of DMAIC ensures that each process that undergoes the transformative efforts in DMAI become institutionalized (i.e., broadly adopted for relevant processes throughout the enterprise). The Control Phase not only incorporates monitoring and improvement mechanisms, but it also ensures that customer feedback and preferences are also included in the continuing evaluation of the value stream.

In recent years, the concept of the High Reliability Organization (HRO) has become increasingly valuable in setting healthcare standards. Simply put, the HRO provides care at consistently high quality and low cost, using many of the tools discussed in this chapter. The value of the HRO concept is evident: unfailing devotion to quality and cost equate to reliable patient outcomes by ensuring that each patient receives the optimum value at each encounter. Lean Six Sigma is ideally suited for developing a HRO, since the key metric Defects per Million Opportunities (DPMO) relates directly to reliability. Although not all attributes of patient encounters yield easily to the DPMO measure, most of the more invasive interventions do indeed have such metrics, such as Central Line Associated Blood Stream Infections, Pressure Ulcer occurrence rates, Ventilator Associated Pneumonia, etc. Progressive healthcare organizations have adopted these metrics as part of their core measurement systems to improve reliability and ensure the best patient outcomes. The Control Phase lays the foundation for the HRO.

Deming also produced 14 principles for quality improvement, termed his "System of Profound Knowledge,"[1] that serve as a useful guide for creation of the cultural framework for the Control Phase:

1. **Create constancy of purpose toward quality improvement of product and service, with the aim of being competitive**–this principle requires that all processes be aligned with the overarching goal of patient safety and quality care.

2. **Adopt the new philosophy of leadership and change for the new economic age**–leaders no longer can be autocratic, but must become coaches and learn to motivate their teams, rather than simply command. Leaders must be as comfortable participating on a team as leading it.

3. **Cease dependence on inspection for quality by building quality into the product in the first place**–as processes are designed or improved, efforts should be directed at reaching and maintaining Six Sigma levels of performance, rather than depending on inspections to identify defects and lead to corrective actions

4. **End the practice of awarding business on the basis of a price tag**–understand and capitalize on relationships with high quality vendors, referral sources, and other resources. As the healthcare industry moves into the era of value-based purchasing (VBP), this principle becomes more important, and many contract relationships will be built on which partners provide the greatest quality, as well as on cost.

5. **Improve constantly and forever the system of production and service, to improve quality and productivity, and thus constantly reduce costs**–interestingly, Deming espoused this idea of creating value in business systems three decades before VBP became a buzzword in health care.

6. **Institute training on the job**–training at the site of work is not a new phenomenon in medicine, as most practitioners are familiar with internships and other arrangements that have been used for centuries to train new generations of practitioners; Deming advocated for similar methods of ongoing training to improve quality. New methods of training in healthcare settings, such as Web-based services, bring education closer to the front line of care.

7. **Institute leadership**–the idea of the "new philosophy of leadership" must be disseminated to the entire leadership team and applied to frontline management, as well as executive management. Supervisors must understand the tenets of teamwork and management by influence, rather than use of coercion to gain team performance.

8. **Drive out fear, so that everyone may work effectively for the company**–this principle relates to several other Deming standards, in that the use of fear to motivate employees is never effective. Deming believed that using fear as a motivator was not only ineffective, but typically counterproductive. Workers who are not motivated to do well, but rather try to find ways of avoiding the wrath of supervisors, will not perform optimally to achieve the goals of the organization.

9. **Break down barriers between departments**–the effects of silos are well known in health care, and one of the greatest challenges in health care today relates to errors produced at transition points between points of care or departments within an organization. Deming saw the need for removing barriers to communication in manufacturing, but those barriers are also critically important in health care as a source for patient safety hazards, increased costs, and lapses in quality.

10. **Eliminate slogans, exhortations, and targets asking for zero defects and new levels of productivity; eliminate work standards (quotas) and management by objective, numbers, and numerical goals; realize that low quality belongs to the system and is beyond the power of the workforce; instead substitute leadership**–Deming referred to many of the common management buzzwords of his era in the 1950s through the 1990s when he taught and published. The major point of this principle is the importance of leadership in shaping performance in an organization. The Control Phase uses numerous approaches to standardize and institutionalize effective change, but without leadership engagement and support, none of these methods will succeed.

11. **Remove barriers that rob workers their right to pride of workmanship by eliminating ratings systems and management by objective**–Abraham Maslow published his hierarchy of needs in the 1950s,[2] and the pinnacle of the hierarchy is self-actualization, a description of an individual achieving his or her full potential.

Deming realized that workers who reached this level of personality development would also achieve their greatest levels of performance, and he asserted that optimizing the worker's engagement in the workplace would improve quality and reduce costs.

12. **Remove barriers that rob people in management and in engineering of their right to pride of workmanship**–one of Deming's pet peeves was personnel rating systems, and this principle was directed at that practice. In a healthcare setting, that issue might entail ranking systems used to rate everything from providers to facilities; these rankings often do not measure appropriate factors related to quality, and having people work solely to improve rankings instead of addressing quality issues that have much greater significance ultimately leads to poorer performance. Focusing on these less relevant issues often removes the pride of workmanship that people, particularly highly educated professionals, feel toward their work.

13. **Institute a vigorous program of education and self-improvement**–Deming advocated continuing education as a way of improving quality, and this philosophy is well established in the healthcare environment. Effective managers find ways of incorporating education and self-improvement programs into the work environment, as reflected in many companies' policies on encouraging employee education through benefits such as tuition assistance and online learning programs.

14. **Put everyone in the company to work to accomplish this transformation**–the role of quality in an organization should be central to everyone's job, not just the task of a quality improvement department. Many healthcare organizations tend to centralize improvement efforts in a single department, without incorporating quality measurement and improvement throughout the enterprise. Deming emphasized the fallacy of this approach and encouraged organizations to move quality out to the entire company.

Deming's 14 principles and System of Profound Knowledge can help any organization, regardless of the industry, structure quality improvement efforts in a cultural framework that engages workers and places the focus on continual improvement. Application of Control Phase tools in a culture based on these principles will create more sustainable improvements and increase the likelihood of long-term success.

# CONTROL PHASE TOOLS

## *Flowcharts*

Once the new process has been defined through the Improve Phase, a new flowchart helps stakeholders understand enhanced procedures and the implications of new policies. Creation of flowcharts and process diagrams is covered in more depth in Chapters 2 and 3, but the use of flowcharts in LSS is a recurring theme, since they convey a wealth of information in a relatively simple diagram. Since the flowchart is a key part of the DMAIC approach, the team should create and maintain the process flow diagram as a core task.

Some specialized variations on the basic flowchart can sometimes communicate important messages to process stakeholders. Two charts in particular are used in LSS projects: the Critical-to-Quality (CTQ) diagrams and the Critical-to-the-Customer (CTC) charts. Some CTQ diagrams are typically in the form of decision trees, such as that shown in **Figure 6-1**, while others might simply highlight certain steps in a basic flowchart as demonstrated in **Figure 6-2**. Each chart has a slightly different function as described in Example 6-1.

---

## Example 6-1 Improving hospital acquired pressure ulcer occurrence rates

Senior managers at CleanDerm Hospital were concerned with the rise in the incidence of hospital acquired pressure ulcers (HAPUs) on the rehab floor. The HAPU rate per 1,000 patient days had risen from 1.4 in Q1 2007 to 2.5 in Q4 2010 as shown in **Table 6-1**.

These rates now exceeded the median benchmarks that the hospital used to assess the quality of care, and so the leadership team commissioned a DMAIC project championed by the vice president of nursing that identified a number of process issues that were effectively reengineered during the Improve Phase. The DMAIC team (named HAPUStop) wanted to succinctly communicate the CTQs to the rehab floor's stakeholders and produced the two diagrams in Figures 6-1 and 6-2. Figure 6-1 quickly describes the new or revised tasks for each stakeholder involved in the patient's care, such as addition of the Braden Scale measurement system for nurses at each daily assessment. Figure 6-2 shows a generic daily care plan with the new PU assessment interventions highlighted as CTQ requirements in the workflow.

**Table 6-1**  HAPU rates per 1,000 patient days at CleanDerm Hospital

| Year | Q1 | Q2 | Q3 | Q4 |
|------|-----|-----|-----|-----|
| 2007 | 1.4 | 1.1 | 1.2 | 1.1 |
| 2008 | 1.7 | 1.9 | 1.9 | 1.8 |
| 2009 | 1.9 | 2.1 | 2.3 | 2.4 |
| 2010 | 2.2 | 2.4 | 2.4 | 2.5 |

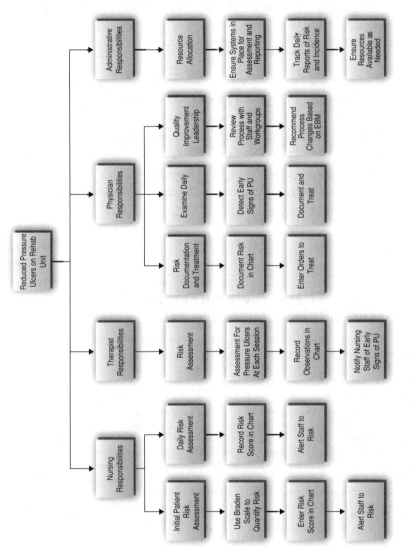

**FIGURE 6-1** Critical to Quality Tree

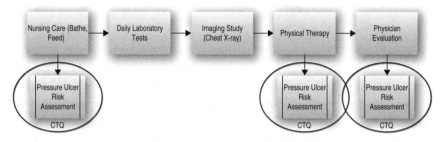

**FIGURE 6-2** CTQ highlights in daily care plan for improving pressure ulcer incidence

Another type of flowchart that is valuable during this phase is the deployment flowchart, as discussed in Chapter 5. The deployment flowchart provides a clear distinction of who is responsible for each task in the newly designed process and helps teams align accountability with individuals and departments. Using the deployment flowchart the team can quickly outline responsibilities and get individuals and departments to "sign off" on the changes, and then use those agreements to ensure that process performance metrics are specifically attributed, rather than being vague and unenforceable.

### Standardization and Institutionalization of Process Changes

The goal of the Control Phase is to guarantee that the gains made in the improvement project are both deployed throughout the organization and sustained over time, and the LSS approach is to standardize the process improvement and institutionalize the process change. Most teams encounter workforce inertia to change that inhibits both of these efforts, and so some specific strategies are necessary to achieve these goals. To begin, it is important to understand these concepts in more detail.

Standardization is one of the "gold chalices" of many businesses, and it has been achieved by some. This concept entails performing a particular process reliably the same way every time the process is run. A rather extreme example of the concept is the assembly line construction of a car part—often performed by machines that maintain strict tolerances based on specific requirements. In health care, more flexibility is generally required, since dealing with human clinical parameters introduces variables that require responses that can be adjusted for variation. For example, the use of standardized protocols for cardiopulmonary resuscitation using Advanced

Cardiac Life Support (ACLS) or Pediatric Advanced Life Support (PALS) protocols provides standard approaches, but the clinical condition and changes in patient status allow adjustment in the application of the protocols to meet patient needs. The processes within each of these protocols are rigorously standardized, thus preventing a number of potential errors, but the application of each process (e.g., administration of epinephrine for specific clinical conditions) is determined based on clinical judgment by the attending provider. Many processes in health care require that level of flexibility, but many more can be standardized to achieve consistency in performance and reduce costly variation.

Nearly all companies have policies and procedures (P&Ps) to standardize behaviors that are essential to organizational performance, as well as ensuring that improvements made during a DMAIC project become part of the organizational routine. Policies are principles, rules, and guidelines that the team creates to codify the improvements realized during a project. Policies are designed to direct all of the activities related to a function or process, and they may include not just the learning from a DMAIC project, but also other tenets from laws, regulations, and standards from accrediting agencies. Every action in a process should relate to one or more of the elements of the policy that governs the process. Procedures emanate directly from policies and are the specific methods employed to actualize policies in day-to-day operations. Most organizations deploy policies and procedures together, to ensure that the policies are actually implemented. Policies are not always a result of a performance improvement project; indeed, policies can be promulgated as noted previously from standards set by accrediting organizations, rules set forth in regulations by state agencies, or laws passed by federal or state legislatures. Additionally, policies are usually formulated to be consistent with the mission, vision, and values of the organization (see **Figure 6-3**). The figure shows that multiple inputs integrate into a policy, which then is used to develop a number of procedures that are translated into even more frontline tools like clinical practice guidelines, standard orders, templates for recording patient documentation, or for templates that can be used in business processes.

Clinical practice guidelines (CPGs) that have become the cornerstone of care management programs to improve quality and reduce cost in the healthcare delivery system. CPGs were defined in the late 1980s by the forerunner of the Agency for Healthcare Research and Quality as "… systematically developed statements to assist practitioner and patient

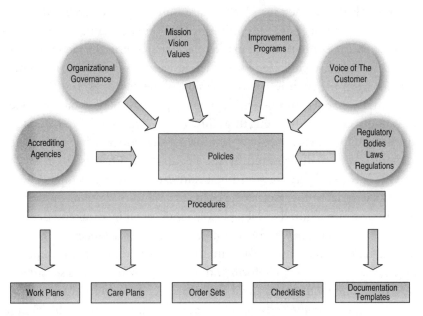

**FIGURE 6-3** Formulation of policies and procedures

decisions about appropriate health care for specific clinical circumstances."[3] Since those early days, CPGs have evolved into valuable tools for standardizing care by providing frontline practitioners with specific recommendations regarding leading practices for patient care. In addition to serving as a decision support tool, CPGs have a number of other purposes:

- Standardization of care to reduce inappropriate variation in medical practice
- Better definition of what specialties are involved in care of clinical conditions and define communication protocols between providers
- Establishment of a basis for comparing current practitioner care patterns with leading practices
- Identification of gaps in care through process and outcome measures to direct continuing professional education
- Increasing the ability to identify resource requirements and more efficiently allocate resources to care processes
- Development of research programs to close knowledge gaps
- Format for decision support in electronic medical record systems

Although the Agency for Health Care Policy and Research (AHCPR) established a robust format for CPGs in 1989, that design is not regularly followed in the contemporary marketplace. The Clinical Practice Guideline Clearinghouse (http://www.guidelines.gov) has CPGs in numerous formats, from the traditional arrangement pioneered by AHCPR to published meta-analyses from scientific medical journals. Payers have changed these tools even further, creating clinical coverage guidelines (CCGs), which are CPGs that are edited to inform practitioners what parts of the guideline are actually covered by the health plan. One useful aspect of the CCGs is the ability for frontline healthcare providers to understand a patient's insurance coverage at the point of care so that the recommendations for care are tailored to each person's individual medical and financial circumstances. This new information resource has introduced the concept of value-based purchasing (VBP) into the doctor-patient relationship, paving the way for healthcare reform and making providers more sensitive to the costs that patients must incur for recommended services.

CPGs have become indispensible tools for improvement throughout the world, and numerous sources for CPGs are available, as indicated in **Table 6-2**. Many provider and payer organizations now use both domestic and international guidelines to formulate care plans that establish the internal standards of care for the enterprise, and then use the care plans to evaluate provider performance and align incentives with leading practices. CPGs thus are applicable to the Control Phase of DMAIC as a tool for both formulating and translating an improvement into a policy that can become part of the operational norm of the organization.

**Table 6-2** Sources of clinical practice guidelines

| Sponsor | Name | Website |
|---|---|---|
| Agency for Healthcare Research and Quality (AHRQ) | National Guideline Clearinghouse | http://www.guideline.gov |
| American College of Physicians (ACP) | ACP Clinical Practice Guidelines | http://www.acponline.org/clinical_information/guidelines/ |
| National Heart Lung and Blood Institute (NHLBI) | NHLBI Clinical Practice Guidelines | http://www.nhlbi.nih.gov/guidelines/index.htm |

## Table 6-2  Sources of clinical practice guidelines (*continued*)

| Sponsor | Name | Website |
|---|---|---|
| Canadian Medical Association | CMA Clinical Practice Guidelines | http://www.cma.ca/clinicalresources/practiceguidelines |
| Haute Autorité de Santé. (French National Authority for Health) | HAS Clinical Guidelines | http://www.has-sante.fr/portail/jcms/c_5443/english?cid=c_5443 |
| Ärtzlichen Zentrums für Qualität in der Medizin (Physicians Center for Medical Quality) | Leitlinien.de | http://www.leitlinien.de/ |
| Istituto Superiore de Sanità (Italian National Institute of Health) | Linee guida nazionali | http://www.snlg-iss.it/home_en# |
| Kwaliteitsinstituut voor de Gezondheidszorg (CBO)– Dutch Institute for Health Improvement | Richtlijnen | http://www.cbo.nl/en/Guidelines/ |
| Scottish Intercollegiate Guidelines Network | SIGN Guidelines | http://www.sign.ac.uk/ |
| National Institute for Health and Clinical Excellence (NICE)– England and Wales | NICE Guidelines | http://www.nice.org.uk/ |
| NHS Evidence– England and Wales | Clinical Knowledge Summaries (CKS) | http://cks.nhs.uk |
| Ministry of Health– Singapore | Clinical Practice Guidelines | http://www.moh.gov.sg/mohcorp/publications.aspx?id=16266 |
| Academy of Medicine –Malaysia | Clinical Practice Guidelines (CPGs) | http://www.acadmed.org.my/index.cfm?&menuid=67 |
| Australian Government Department of Health and Ageing | Treatment and Techniques | http://www.health.gov.au/internet/main/publishing.nsf/Content/Treatment+and+Techniques-1 |
| Medical Journal of Australia | Guidelines, position statements, and consensus statements | http://www.mja.com.au/public/guides/guides.html |
| New Zealand Guidelines Group | Guidelines | http://www.nzgg.org.nz/index.cfm |

Another important tool used in standardization is the checklist. The value of checklists in healthcare has recently become the subject of a number of publications,[4] but the use of checklists for quality assurance has a long history. Checklists provide an ordered sequence of steps in a process, and so they fit well in the Control Phase of DMAIC. Most checklists for processes include short descriptions of the steps or at least a reference to descriptions in an underlying policy and/or procedure. An example checklist for a patient visit in a medical office is shown in **Figure 6-4**. Note that the checklist is divided into tasks by the individual performing the task (registration, nurse, physician), and each task connotes a step in the office visit process. Examples of other checklists are listed in the Other Resources section of this chapter.

Institutionalizing change in the Control Phase requires several steps that relate to the workforce, in addition to the tools that are used to systematize the changes. The importance of leadership support in the Control Phase, particularly for making needed changes permanent for the organization, cannot be overemphasized. Resource reallocation can often be met with resistance among those whose current work is affected, and in particular for managers who see their departments realigned to the new processes. Thus, senior leaders must support the changes, both verbally and through resource assignment and incentive realignment. Individual workplace plans will likely need to be changed to conform to the new process, and the ability of workforce members to maintain their productivity in the new environment (especially if productivity is linked to pay) becomes a crucial success factor. Example 6-2 describes a common scenario in a healthcare system that is implementing and electronic medical record (EMR).

---

## Example 6-2 Implementation of an EMR at a medical center

Dr. Bill Brickwell, the Chief Medical Information Officer at a multihospital medical center, has the responsibility to implement the organization's EMR, including computerized provider order entry (CPOE) and physician documentation, at three of the organization's hospitals to demonstrate that the system was feasible for the rest of the system. The EMR is to be used in both the inpatient and outpatient areas, and so Bill commissioned Six Sigma design groups for each venue. After reviewing the process changes in each of the two areas, Bill assembled a task force of physicians to review the plans and begin to test the system in a pilot-testing environment. Although the system performed well in the inpatient setting, physicians found that productivity in the outpatient department plummeted by nearly 20%, leading to a "mini-revolution" among the doctors, since they had incentives based on patient visit volume. The DMAIC outpatient team reviewed the workflow process for using the EMR for documentation and CPOE, and a few changes were made to the data entry sequence, but the physicians' productivity did not improve. The team was aware of the productivity "hits" that occur with EMR implementation that were found during the Define Phase during a literature search, but they had not anticipated the level of physician push back. The literature sources indicated that physician productivity usually returned to normal levels at about six months post-implementation, and so Dr. Brickwell worked with the CMO and CFO to redesign the physicians' incentive program for the six-month "phase-in" period. The new incentive program reset patient visit work relative value units (WRVUs) to a lower rate from the start of EMR deployment, with gradually increasing WRVU levels over the next six months. At six months post-implementation, incentive WRVU levels returned to their pre-implementation levels. The staff physicians found this solution equitable, and the "mini-revolution" subsided quickly.

Example 6-2 is explication of the need for senior management engagement in the DMAIC program. Without the ability to change the financial arrangements quickly, the implementation of the outpatient EMR would likely have been delayed, if not an outright failure.

Despite best efforts at standardization, many process improvements will meet challenges during the Control Phase because the underlying structure and/or workforce knowledge have not changed. In these cases, staff members will typically develop "workarounds" that try to adjust to the new process without changing fundamental behavior. This phenomenon is predictable from the quality improvement experience in any number of industries and the observation that every worker tries to optimize performance in the environment in which they work. If a new process is not conducive to continued productivity, then workers typically find ways around the required process steps to make the process functional for their own circumstance. The goal of standardization is lost in these situations, and so the Control Phase plan must include tracking and monitoring systems that detect these anomalous behaviors and allow intervention with the process user. In most cases, workarounds are the result of incomplete understanding of the new process due to ineffective training, but sometimes the workaround can indicate an opportunity for improvement. Thus, workarounds should not be summarily dismissed, but rather examined as opportunities. The key underlying assumption, however, should not be that a worker is being recalcitrant, but rather that either the process is still flawed or the implementation and training were not adequate.

---

**Patient Visit Checklist**
**ABC Clinic**


Patient Name: _____     Visit Date: _____

### Registration
- [ ] Patient in billing system
- [ ] Patient information updated in billing system
- [ ] Guarantor in billing system
- [ ] Guarantor information updated in billing system
- [ ] Insurance information updated in billing system
- [ ] Patient information in EMR

### Nurse
- [ ] Patient vital signs entered into EMR (height, weight, BP, OFC)
- [ ] Patient chief complaint entered into EMR
- [ ] Patient interim history entered into EMR
- [ ] Appropriate care plan selected
- [ ] Medication history entered into EMR

### Physician
- [ ] Physician review and update to interim history
- [ ] Physician review of vital signs
- [ ] Physician review of medication list
- [ ] Physician check off on care plan
- [ ] Physician physical exam performed and recorded
- [ ] Physician diagnostic recommendations entered into EMR
- [ ] Physician therapeutic recommendations entered into EMR
- [ ] Physician medication prescriptions entered into EMR

### Nurse
- [ ] Physician diagnostic recommendations reviewed
- [ ] Physician therapeutic recommendations reviewed
- [ ] Physician medication prescriptions reviewed
- [ ] Recommendations and prescriptions reconciled with care plan
- [ ] Medication reconciliation performed
- [ ] Patient educational materials selected
- [ ] Patient educational materials reviewed with patient/caretaker

### Registration
- [ ] Patient/guarantor visit reviewed in billing system
- [ ] Copays/deductibles collected or arranged
- [ ] Referral appointment(s) made
- [ ] Follow up appointment made
- [ ] Ensure checklist completed

---

**FIGURE 6-4** Checklist for patient office visit

## Training Plans and Programs

Ensuring that every relevant stakeholder understands the improvements planned for a process is a key part of the Control Phase. The training program should be tailored to stakeholder needs, and so it might consist of several modules that can be parsed out to subgroups of stakeholders based on their specific needs. In most cases, training program development starts at the end of the Improve Phase as an intervention is piloted and lessons learned about implementation. The program is then finalized and "polished" during the Control Phase and becomes a long-term strategy for ensuring adherence to the improvement plan.

A key component of the training program involves communicating the training to all employees who might be touched by the process. The format of the training program may vary, but the content should include:

- **Document history**–a table at the beginning of the document that details dates and times that versions have been published; the last entry in the table is the most recent version with the time and date that it was published.
- **Approvals**–a table at the beginning of the document with signatures, date signed, and printed name of everyone whose approval is required for the training plan
- **Table of contents**–list of sections and page numbers of the content of the training program
- **Purpose of the document**
  - Overall training scope and strategy
  - Training requirements
  - Proposed training sessions
  - Required training materials
  - Facilities.
  - The plan is developed during the Planning Phase. The project manager is responsible for developing and distributing the training plan to all team members, project sponsors and to the supervisors of the target training audience.
- **Acronyms and abbreviations**–a table of acronyms and abbreviations used throughout the document
- **Executive summary**–short description of the contents of the program for use by senior leaders to quickly understand the program and its stakeholders

- **Scope**
  - Staff members affected by the program
  - Departments to be included in the training
  - Duration of the program
  - Number of training sessions planned
- **Background**
  - Brief description of the project that led to the program
  - Overview of the content
  - Expected results from training and improvement programs
- **Strategy**
  - Approach to training (e.g., train the trainers)
  - Grouping of trainees (e.g., IT, nurses, physicians)
  - Phased training at different stages of implementation
  - Training developed in house or purchased courses
- **Training requirements**
  - General background of training participants (e.g., educational level, job category)
  - Specific training interventions for specific individuals or positions
  - Time frame for training
- **Roles and responsibilities**
  - Roles and responsibilities of training staff (e.g., management of content development, implementation, media management)
  - Course presenters
  - Instructors
  - Resource staff
  - Consultants
  - Roles and responsibilities
- **Training sessions**–for each session:
  - Outline of content
  - Instructor
  - Course objectives
  - Duration
  - Mode of instruction (e.g., hands-on, self-learning, online, face-to-face)
  - Medium (e.g., online, transportable media, synchronous, asynchronous)
- **Training evaluation**
  - Evaluation approaches and tools
  - Forms

- Data collection
- Data analysis and reports
- Use of feedback to improve course(s)
- **Constraints and limitations**
  - Dependencies on other companies, staff members, departments
  - Limitations that could slow project (e.g., funding, instructor availability)
- **Training materials**
  - Handouts
  - Slides
  - Materials for demonstrations
  - Workbooks
  - Manuals
  - Electronic decision support materials
  - Software
  - Hardware
  - Instructor guide
- **Plan for training material revisions**
  - Details of methods by which training materials are revised and updated as the program matures
  - Training team involvement with updates
- **Facilities**
  - Computers and other equipment required by each trainee
  - Computers and other equipment required by instructors
  - Software required by trainees
  - Software required by instructors
  - Locations of training
- **Glossary**
  - Technical terms
  - Trade terms
  - Department or company-specific terms

Most organizations create a template for training program development that meets the requirements set by senior managers or training facility managers, and each program is then cataloged in the organization's knowledge base.

It is important to ensure that the training program addresses the issues needed by the workforce to properly implement the process improvement. Nearly every training program has an evaluation of the training, but use of an evaluation model like the Kirkpatrick Learning and Training Evaluation Theory,[5] which provides a deeper understanding of the efficacy of a training program as shown in **Table 6-3.**

The Kirkpatrick model requires not just evaluation of the training program, but also the effect that the training had on both individual performance and organizational performance. Although the third and fourth levels of evaluation become increasingly difficult to measure, the goal of

**Table 6-3** Kirkpatrick Learning and Training Evaluation Model

| Level | Measurement | Description | Example tools | Comments |
|-------|-------------|-------------|---------------|----------|
| 1 | Reaction | How trainees felt about the training experience (e.g., instructor effectiveness, materials for the course, facilities, take-home work) | Feedback forms Verbal feedback to staff and instructors | Easy to obtain and analyze Usually not expensive |
| 2 | Learning | Measurement of increase in knowledge caused by the course or training | Before and after tests Interviews, observation of skills | Relatively straightforward to administer Difficult for complex educational programs |
| 3 | Behavior | Extent of application of learning on the job after the training | Observation/ interview by trainers or supervisors Metrics to assess performance before and after training Trends in metrics over time | More difficult to administer and sustain after training Best done with objective measures, rather than subjective observations |
| 4 | Results | Effect on the business or clinical performance | Metrics in use by management team to measure organizational performance | Multiple confounding factors make direct attribution to individual effort and/or training difficult to discern |

Data from: Kirkpatrick D, Kirkpatrick J. (2005). *Transferring learning to behavior: Using the four levels to improve performance.* Berrett-Koehler Publishers, San Francisco, CA. Table is Dr. Lighter's creation.

training to influence individual and organizational performance is frequently measurable and very useful to determine if the training program is worth the expense and effort.

## Monitoring Plans

The monitoring plan is another deliverable from the Control Phase. The business and clinical environment in health care changes constantly, and once an improvement is deployed, almost inevitably the world in which the process is operating changes, affecting performance. Without some way of monitoring those changes, it is difficult to determine if the process improvement remains viable. As noted previously, one potential pitfall is the worker who finds workarounds to process steps that also could decrease process performance. Thus, an effective monitoring plan is necessary to not only determine if the desired improvements in performance are sustained, but the plan should also contain metrics that aid in troubleshooting lagging process execution.

The monitoring plan should contain the following elements:

- Clear identification of the process being monitored
- Process owners and stakeholders
- Critical-to-Quality (CTQ) measures identified in the Define Phase
- Performance targets and benchmarks
  - Exemplary performance levels indicating opportunity for recognition
  - Red flags for poor performance indicating a need to intervene aggressively
- Process metrics–measures that monitor key process steps
- Outcome metrics–including CTQ measures, but also other metrics that indicate that the process output is achieving goals
- Intervention plan for varying levels of declining performance
  - Education programs
  - Root Cause Analysis
  - FMEA
  - DMAIC team
- Tools used for monitoring
  - Trend charts
  - Control charts
  - Dashboards with red-yellow-green indicators
- Process for reevaluating the monitoring system for adequacy

A monitoring plan, combined with the training program, is one of the key deliverables from the Control Phase. Use of the plan ensures that the process improvement is not only implemented effectively, but it also is sustainable, since the improvements that might have been so difficult to achieve are being actively watched to avoid regressing to prior levels of poor performance.

### Poka Yoke

Poka yoke is a Japanese term used in the Lean Management System that is translated as "mistake proofing." The goal in a Lean Six Sigma production system is to recognize errors as soon as they occur in the process so that they may be corrected before they propagate. The purpose of poka yoke techniques and tools is to ensure that conditions are set in the process environment to avoid errors, rather than correcting them. The poka yoke concept is behind myriad improvements in the healthcare industry, from tall man characters on pharmaceutical labels to different colored gas tanks for anesthesia machines to different types of wall connectors for oxygen and suction in hospitals. A detailed discussion of mistake proofing can be found in John Grout's important text on mistake-proofing in health care.[6]

Grout describes human responses to action as divided into two steps: 1) understanding the intent of the action and 2) performing the action based on the intent. Errors occur when humans do not understand the intent and do not perform the action properly or at all, or when the intention is understood but the action is executed improperly. Although mistake proofing is possible in either situation, it is typically applied when the intent is known and execution fails. Mistake proofing relies on other techniques like FMEA (Chapter 3) and RCA (Chapter 4) to identify the underlying issues that have led to an error, and then implementing solutions is usually done in a systematic way to optimize improvement yields. A mistake proofing effort usually proceeds as noted in **Table 6-4**.

Poka yoke approaches anticipate errors and provide techniques to detect them early or prevent them altogether, and mistake-proofing efforts are often divided into prevention and detection approaches. Several of these approaches have been applied in health care to reduce errors and improve safety, including:

- **Education and training**–used mainly for prevention, the goal of training is to ensure competence and decrease the probability of errors. On the other hand, training can also increase alertness for finding errors after they have occurred.

**Table 6-4**  Procedure for mistake proofing

| Step | Description | Deliverable | Comment |
|---|---|---|---|
| 1 | Use data to select a process that has a high level or probability of error | Process selected, target errors identified | • Sources of data include scorecards, regulatory reports, accreditation reviews, new requirements for compliance, customer complaints |
| 2 | Determine stakeholders and/or departments involved in the process and select cross-functional team | Cross functional team identified representing all relevant stakeholders | • Most processes affect nearly all departments, but the most relevant stakeholders are those who control inputs, perform the process, and directly use process outputs |
| 3 | Convene stakeholders in Kaizen event to perform an FMEA or RCA | FMEA or RCA results that indicate one or more process steps, equipment malfunctions, or design elements that require mistake proofing | • Results should indicate the point in the process at which an intervention is needed, either though redesign or through equipment modifications |
| 4 | Evaluate the identified issue(s) for mistake proofing interventions | Mistake proofing intervention(s) | • Brainstorming is the favored approach in most cases of mistake proofing, but in some cases, specific engineering skills might be needed, requiring manufacturer participation in the effort<br>• Interventions should be<br>　• Inexpensive<br>　• Based on logic and common sense<br>　• Weighted toward recommendations from frontline workers<br>　• Directed at eliminating the occurrence or detecting the problem as early in the process as possible |
| 5 | Pilot test the mistake proofing intervention | Results of pilot study testing interventions | • Cost should be evaluated along with efficacy of the intervention<br>• Pilot testing should last long enough to ensure that an error has been prevented |
| 6 | Effective changes in the pilot test are deployed to the rest of the organization | Process/equipment changes are disseminated throughout the organization to affected departments | • Deployment may require significant investment, so a plan for the deployment may need to include financial data, as well as procedural information |

- **"Natural mapping"**–this approach strives to prevent errors by placing process or equipment controls close to the affected process step or piece of equipment. For example, anesthesia machines place anesthesia controls very close to their respective gas cylinders to allow rapid checking of the gas being delivered to the patient.
- **Forcing functions**–create process steps or equipment usage patterns that require the process to proceed in only one (correct) way. For example, some e-prescription programs notify physicians when a medication being requested interacts adversely with another medication or food that the patient is currently taking. Physicians may override the alert in some situations, but where a clear danger exists, the request is referred to a pharmacist for further review and intervention.
- **6S orderliness**–conduct a 6S exercise (Chapter 5) periodically to ensure that the workplace is orderly and that necessary equipment and supplies are readily visible.
- **Visibility**–ensure that process steps, measures, supplies, or equipment parts are easily visible to workers who need the information or materials to perform their work. Kanban is a method of lean management that promotes the use of visual cues and signage to reduce errors and bring information to the point of work.
- **Feedback loops**–ensure that each critical step in a process has metrics that are fed back to the process user in sufficient time to foresee and prevent an error. For example, an alarm that sounds when an IV solution is completely infused.

In the context of the Control Phase, poka yoke is an important method of setting up control systems to function in only one way. If an improvement is to be successfully deployed and sustained, it must be implemented in a manner consistent with the way it was developed during the Improve Phase. Applying the tenets of mistake proofing can help ensure success of the implementation, as demonstrated in Example 6-3.

---

## Example 6-3 Applying poka yoke to the Control Phase

The improvement team at FASTLabs had met its goal during the pilot test in the Improve Phase of their DMAIC project. They had reduced the average time required to perform a Complete Blood Count to 8 minutes from 25 minutes and reduced the error rate from $3.5\sigma$ to $4.2\sigma$. The improvement process included using 6S to rearrange the lab equipment and reorganizing the supply drawers so that older supplies were in front (thus removed first). The 6S approach was also used to place the three required test supply elements into kits so that lab techs did not need to search for one of the components. The team also applied Kanban by placing an "out of stock card" in the supply cabinet so that critical supplies were always restocked in a timely manner. Finally, the team used feedback loops to ensure that the equipment was properly calibrated by placing the control testing report sheets directly beside the Coulter counter so that the tech could be sure that the machine had been recently calibrated. To ensure that deployment of the process improvements was equally successful, the team created a training plan, and included forcing functions to ensure that the flow of lab specimens followed the ideal approach that was demonstrated in the pilot test. For example, the team placed the supply kits in a drawer in the lab directly adjacent to the automated blood analysis machine and assigned one lab support person to inspect the inventory of supplies daily, recording findings on a log that folded out from the drawer and could easily be checked by lab techs or the lab supervisor. The lab supervisor made review of the supplies log a part of his daily routine (a key component of the Control Phase audit plan), and if the checklist was not completed, he ensured that the lab support person stocked the supply drawer quickly. The lab supervisor also made the lab support person accountable for ensuring that the supply inventory was checked and restocked as needed, and also responsible for ensuring that the CBC kits were always available.

Mistake proofing has numerous applications in health care, but it can also be an important part of the Control Phase. Using the tools of poka yoke, the DMAIC team can ensure that the improvements piloted during the Improve Phase are implemented effectively.

## Audit Plans

Although Deming's goal of eliminating inspections through quality assurance is laudable, the reality of the regulatory and legal environment of health care simply do not allow for elimination of all inspections. Thus, an audit plan should be part of the Control Phase of each DMAIC project, not just to ensure that the gains from the Improve Phase are sustained, but often also to meet regulatory and compliance requirements. An audit plan provides a systematic method of ensuring that improvements are sustained, as well as compliant with the regulatory, accreditation, and legal requirements that healthcare organizations must meet. In the healthcare industry, audit plans are often called "surveillance," which connotes oversight and measurement of ongoing operations for specific events or trends that connote a deviation from expected performance. One common type of healthcare surveillance targets infection control, and infection control professionals in health systems track the types of infections that are occurring in the system and the community, including issues of resistance to antimicrobial drugs and types of hosts (patients) in whom the infections are occurring. Infection control surveillance systems are important for early detection of new infectious agents, drug resistance patterns, and quality of care issues related to antiseptic processes in the healthcare organization. Audit plans in other industries follow a similar pattern and may be subject to other regulatory frameworks (e.g., protocols established by the International Organization for Standardization, www.iso.org).

An audit plan must start with a standard or criteria used for comparison. Process audits might identify and compare measures that quantify procedural steps or a similar process benchmark from either the healthcare or other industry. For example, some hospitals now benchmark their food services against those of Baldrige Performance Excellence Program recipient hotel chain Ritz Carlton. Process metrics like delivery time can be gauged for determining process performance and compared to world-class performance. Safety audits often start with safety rules and regulations, which may come from internal standards, or standards from organizations like The Joint Commission or federal regulatory agencies. Outcomes of care, like surgical site infections or mortality after myocardial infarction, are also typically tracked as part of a Control Phase audit plan.

The audit plan outlines five phases:

1. **Audit planning**
   a. Auditor/audit team's preparation phase
   b. Rules to be used in the audit process are identified
   c. Auditors trained in the meaning of the rules and what to observe during the audit
   d. Auditors trained how to complete the reporting template
   e. Where necessary, auditors are certified to perform the audit
   f. Audit is scheduled with affected department/process owner
2. **Audit performance**
   a. Auditors review documents and visit site to make observations
   b. Audited process owner and stakeholders interviewed
   c. Qualitative and quantitative data collected

3. **Audit reporting**
   a. Draft report created with scope, activities, and results
   b. Recommendations for improvement
   c. Preventive actions needed to improve safety
4. **Audit closure**
   a. Delivery of report to process owner
   b. Discussion and explanation of findings
5. **Corrective Action Plan**
   a. Work with process owner and stakeholders to develop plan to remediate audit findings

The audit plan typically describes an internal audit program (i.e., one that is conducted by the organization's staff), but in some cases, external audits might be necessary, as well. For example, if the process has implications for compliance, it might be advantageous to have someone from outside the organization to provide a more objective review than having a coworker conduct the audit.

The task of auditing is important, since the goal of the audit is not to find fault, but rather to identify opportunities for improvement and rectify issues that can lead to inefficiencies and potential problems with patient safety. The audit process depends on a collegial approach, as well as effective preparation to ensure a comprehensive assessment. An audit should be fact based, using data where possible and avoiding conjecture. Additionally, the record of the audit should be clear and unequivocal in the observations made so that the recommendations are unambiguous. The auditor's role is usually highly valued if done properly, but the auditor also gains a great deal in the process, too. Auditors often learn a great deal about the organization, too, and so service in an auditing position has benefits that outweigh the work effort.

## Control Charts

These seminal tools constitute a theme throughout DMAIC and are described in depth in Chapter 3. Nowhere, however, is the control chart more valuable than for the Control Phase. One of the famous dicta of quality improvement is "if it's not measured, it's not managed." During the Control Phase, that principle becomes an axiom that underpins all of the efforts to sustain the improvement. Recall that control charts provide information about the trend of a process measure plotted on a graph with the mean and control limits at ±3 sigma levels to differentiate common cause variation from special cause variation. Control charts are especially helpful during the Control Phase because they are helpful for identifying process measure points that are out of control, but these charts also display the trend of the process measure as well.

Clinical applications of control charts to monitor health processes are subject to factors that are not extant in typical industrial uses. Since some clinical processes involve infectious diseases that have seasonal cycles, the data will require adjustment for seasonal variation. For example, using a control chart to monitor the effects of interventions for influenza prevention will require methods to address the cyclical nature of influenza infection in the population, including regional variation. Without these adjustments, a peak in the incidence of influenza may constitute a special cause point, when in fact it is a common cause point. Seasonal adjustments of the data before plotting the control chart helps avoid these Type I (false positive) errors. This approach is helpful in ensuring that seasonal trends are accounted for as the data are analyzed for special causes. Seasonal adjustment of the data is based on the configuration of the data set– e.g., if there is no other apparent trend (flat trend) or if there is also an apparent trend in the data (up-trend or down-trend). Example 6-4 provides an example of a flat trend seasonal adjustment.

## Example 6-4 Seasonal adjustment of influenza trend data

NoFlu Clinic has prided itself with its influenza prevention program for the past three years, and they decided to begin tracking the data using a control chart. The team reviewed the data from the prior five calendar years and produced the graph shown in **Figure 6-5**. Note that the graph indicates seasonal variation in the incidence of influenza cases, with peaks in the first and fourth quarters and troughs in the second and third quarters. Additionally, the trend line drawn through the data indicates a relatively flat trend.

The team also graphed the data and produced the XmR chart shown in **Figure 6-6**. Recall that XmR SPC analysis produces two control charts, one for the actual data and the other for the calculated moving range to determine if the control chart meets the criteria for this type of chart. Note that for the R-chart plot (nonseasonally adjusted data R-chart), a characteristic "saw tooth" pattern is evident, indicating that the pattern of the moving range values indicates a special cause (the seasonality of the data).

Thus, a seasonal adjustment was applied to the data using the approach outlined in **Table 6-5**, and the seasonally adjusted data were subjected to XmR analysis, leading to the graphs in **Figure 6-7**.

Neither of the SPC charts for the seasonally-adjusted data indicate special cause points.

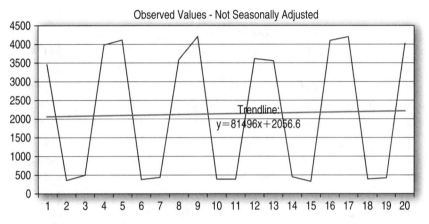

**FIGURE 6-5**  Observed reported influenza cases for NoFlu Clinic

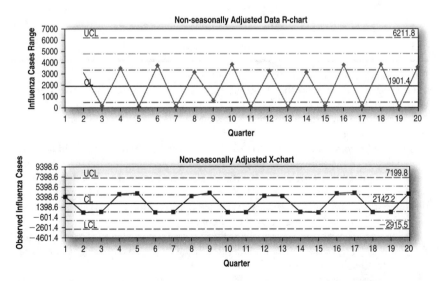

**FIGURE 6-6**  Control chart of the unadjusted data for NoFlu Clinic

**Table 6-5** Procedure for seasonal adjustment of influenza data for NoFlu Clinic

| Year | Quarter | Observed | Trend | Residual | Seasonal factor | Seasonally adjusted series |
|------|---------|----------|-------|----------|-----------------|---------------------------|
| 1 | 1 | 3452 | 2142.15 | 1309.85 | 1788.183 | 1663.8 |
| 1 | 2 | 346 | 2142.15 | −1796.15 | −1773.15 | 2119.2 |
| 1 | 3 | 483 | 2142.15 | −1659.15 | −1707.48 | 2190.5 |
| 1 | 4 | 3984 | 2142.15 | 1841.85 | 1584.85 | 2399.2 |
| 2 | 1 | 4120 | 2142.15 | 1977.85 | 1788.183 | 2331.8 |
| 2 | 2 | 376 | 2142.15 | −1766.15 | −1773.15 | 2149.2 |
| 2 | 3 | 429 | 2142.15 | −1713.15 | −1707.48 | 2136.5 |
| 2 | 4 | 3583 | 2142.15 | 1440.85 | 1584.85 | 1998.2 |
| 3 | 1 | 4219 | 2142.15 | 2076.85 | 1788.183 | 2430.8 |
| 3 | 2 | 385 | 2142.15 | −1757.15 | −1773.15 | 2158.2 |
| 3 | 3 | 392 | 2142.15 | −1750.15 | −1707.48 | 2099.5 |
| 3 | 4 | 3614 | 2142.15 | 1471.85 | 1584.85 | 2029.2 |
| 4 | 1 | 3568 | 2142.15 | 1425.85 | 1788.183 | 1779.8 |
| 4 | 2 | 439 | 2142.15 | −1703.15 | −1773.15 | 2212.2 |
| 4 | 3 | 326 | 2142.15 | −1816.15 | −1707.48 | 2033.5 |
| 4 | 4 | 4103 | 2142.15 | 1960.85 | 1584.85 | 2518.2 |
| 5 | 1 | 4209 | 2142.15 | 2066.85 | 1788.183 | 2420.8 |
| 5 | 2 | 396 | 2142.15 | −1746.15 | −1773.15 | 2169.2 |
| 5 | 3 | 411 | 2142.15 | −1731.15 | −1707.48 | 2118.5 |
| 5 | 4 | 4008 | 2142.15 | 1865.85 | 1584.85 | 2423.2 |

Procedure for calculating seasonally adjusted data series:
1. Calculate the average for the Observed data series, which becomes the trend (in this example, Trend = 2142.15)
2. Subtract the Trend from each Observed value to produce the Residual value (Residual = Observed − Trend)
3. Seasonal Factors are calculated for each quarter as the average of the residuals for each quarter. Thus, all five of the Quarter 1 values are averaged to yield the Seasonal Factor for Quarter 1, all five of the Quarter 2 values are averaged to produce the Seasonal Factor for Quarter 2, etc. The Seasonal Factors are constant for each quarter throughout the data set, so the Seasonal Factor value for Quarter 1 is reproduced for each Quarter 1 entry in the Seasonal Factor column.
4. The Seasonally Adjusted Series is then calculated by subtracting the Seasonal Factor for each quarter from the corresponding value in the Observed data series to produce Seasonally Adjusted Series (Seasonally Adjusted Series Data Point = Observed − Seasonal Factor). For example, for Quarter 1 in Year 1, the Seasonally Adjusted Series Data Point = 3452 − 1788.183 = 1663.8

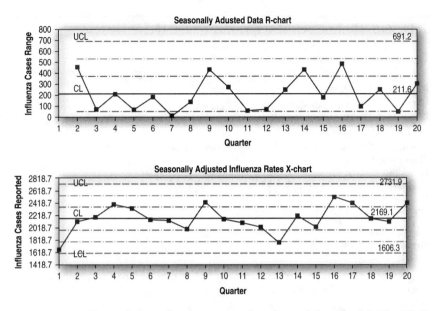

**FIGURE 6-7** Control chart for the seasonally adjusted data for NoFlu Clinic

Another important issue that arises in clinical data tracking using control charts occurs because the populations that are being monitored for improvement initiatives may be sufficiently heterogeneous to require risk adjustment. For example, the population managed by the NoFlu Clinic in Example 6-4 likely consists of smokers and nonsmokers, and since smokers have a higher probability of contracting respiratory illnesses, the data may be adjusted for smoking status. The topic of clinical risk adjustment is complex, and a number of excellent resources provide details (see Other Resources). Risk adjustment has been most frequently applied to payment methods using claims data as demonstrated in Example 6-5, but the approach is being leveraged for making quality improvement initiatives more effective, as well. A number of risk adjustment models have been developed over the past three decades, and some of these models are listed in **Table 6-6**.

**Table 6-6** Healthcare risk adjustment models

| Model | Description |
|---|---|
| Adjusted Clinical Groups (ACGs) | • Morbidity-based ACG categories<br>• Disease-specific Expanded Diagnosis Clusters (EDCs); and diagnostic indicators predict future inpatient care, especially for medically frail |
| Chronic Illness and Disability Payment System (CDPS) | • Diagnosis-based risk assessment model for use with Medicaid populations<br>• Assigns each member to one or more of 67 possible medical condition categories based on diagnosis codes<br>• Subjects also assigned to age/gender category |
| Clinical Risk Grouping (CRG) | • 3M proprietary product<br>• CRG risk groups based on clinical criteria |
| Diagnostic Cost Groups (DCGs) | • Model predicts the total medical cost for each patient based upon the HCC and the age/gender category<br>• DxGroups are used to build DCG models<br>• Diagnosis codes are grouped into 781 clinically homogeneous groups (DxGroups)<br>• DxGroups are further mapped into 184 hierarchical condition categories<br>• Each subject is also assigned to one of 32 age/gender categories |
| Episode Risk Groups (ERGs) | • Based on Episode Treatment Groups (ETGs)<br>• Model assigns each member to one or more of the 120 possible episode risk groups based on ICD and CPT data<br>• Information from both medical and pharmacy claims |
| Impact Pro (Ingenix) | • Groups claims into unique episodes of care and other diagnosis-based Impact Clinical Categories (ICCs)<br>• ICCs describe a subject's observed mix of diseases and conditions, with co-morbidities and complications<br>• ICCs grouped into homogenous risk categories ("base-markers")<br>• Patient may be grouped into one or more base-markers and one demographic marker |
| MEDai. | • Predictions by patient made using combination of clinical factors<br>  • Disease episodes (Symmetry ETGs)<br>  • Drug categories<br>  • Age<br>  • Gender<br>  • Insurance type<br>  • Other risk markers (e.g., timing and frequency of treatment or diagnosis) |

**Table 6-6** Healthcare risk adjustment models (*continued*)

| Model | Description |
|---|---|
| MedicaidRx | • Assigns each member to one or more of 45 medical condition categories based on prescription drug use<br>• Assigns each member to one of 11 age/gender categories<br>• Model predicts the overall medical costs for each member with separate sets of risk weights for adults and children |
| Pharmacy Risk Groups (PRGs) | • Based solely on prescriptions<br>• Maps each NDC to a Pharmacy Risk Group (PRG)<br>• Risk score based on patient's age, gender, and PRG category |
| RxGroups | • Pharmacy-based risk assessment model<br>• Classifies NDCs into 164 mutually exclusive categories (called RxGroups) based on drug's therapeutic indication<br>• Predicts total medical cost based on RxGroups and age/gender category |
| DxCG Underwriting Model, RiskSmart | • Accommodates claims run-out (lag between when service is provided and when claim is adjudicated) to make data more accurate by including six month lag between baseline period and prediction period<br>• Used primarily for underwriting employer groups<br>• Model uses HCCs, disease interactions, age/gender categories and a prior cost variable to predict future medical costs |

# Example 6-5 CMS use of risk adjustment for Medicare Advantage managed care plans

The Centers for Medicare and Medicaid Services (CMS) implemented a risk adjustment model, Hierarchical Condition Categories (HCC), in 2004 that adjusts Medicare capitation payments to Medicare Advantage (MA) healthcare plans to accommodate health expenditure risk of MA enrollees. The goal of the HCC framework has been to ensure that MA plans receive adequate payments to cover the costs of beneficiaries who have higher utilization due to certain illnesses or chronic conditions. Thus, MA plans that enroll healthier members are paid less than those that have sicker members. Sample sizes of over one million in each category were used to establish the risk groupings, and cost data are used to determine relative risk in each category. The model is designed to explain variation at the HCC group level, not at the individual level. The CMS-HCC model uses demographic information (age, sex, Medicaid dual eligibility, disability status) and a profile of major medical conditions in a base year calculation to predict Medicare expenditures in the next year. The Condition Categories are arranged into hierarchies so that individual classifications can be made at the highest possible levels. Each beneficiary in a Medicare Advantage plan is classified using these hierarchies, and capitation payments to MA plans are calculated on the financial amounts allocated to each Condition Category. According to the 2010 Patient Protection and Affordability Act (PPACA), this risk adjustment schema will be applied to the newer payment approaches being deployed, such as bundled payments and Accountable Care Organizations.

The selection of a risk adjustment model depends on a number of factors, including:

- **Affordability and ease of use of the software**–some programs are expensive and require programming skills that create ongoing operational expenses that make the approach less desirable. Proprietary models often fail this test.
- **Population to be analyzed**–models must be matched as closely as possible to populations used to formulate the model.
- **Ease of understanding of the model and reports**–the model should be intuitive to those using the data, and reports should be clear and easy to analyze.
- **Data quality and access, ability to analyze incomplete or imperfect data sets**–rarely are data sets complete, and the system should have built in methods to handle incomplete data sets and the ability to validate questionable data.
- **Integration of clinical and financial results**–value-based purchasing is becoming the key way of evaluating healthcare organizations, and so the ability to integrate clinical and financial results into the model is preferred.
- **Use of the output (e.g., provider payments, underwriting, case and care management)**–models tend to have predictive value for specific outputs, and so the required output must be considered as the model is selected.
- **Reliability of the model across populations, sites of care, geographic locations**–risk adjustment models must accommodate multiple strata within a population, as well as regional differences in patterns of care.
- **Susceptibility of the model to aberrations in the data (e.g., coding abnormalities)**–desirable models have the ability to detect data abnormalities (e.g., improper coding and other errors).

Many of the risk adjustment models are based on financial data, since insurance claims are among the most readily available information that includes both clinical (ICD and CPT coded) and financial data. A number of clinical risk adjustment systems have been devised, as well, but in most cases these models tend to be for specific populations, such as the Acute Physiology and Chronic Health Evaluation (APACHE IV), Simplified

Acute Physiology Score (SAPS II), and the Mortality Probability Model (MPM III) models for ICU patients[7] and similar risk adjustment systems applied to neonatal intensive care units (NICUs).[8] Although claims data are sometimes used for clinical risk adjustment, this approach is fraught with potential errors due to coding inaccuracy and lack of patient specific physiologic parameters.[9]

Administrative risk adjustment is widely deployed among payers in the healthcare industry, but the use of clinical risk adjustment is expected to grow as more clinical data becomes available in electronic medical records. Control Phase monitoring of clinical improvements will benefit greatly from these more accurate statistical adjustments to clinical models.

### Process Sigma Level

The concept of process sigma was originally discussed in Chapter 3, and the metric is particularly germane for the Control Phase. Recall that the process sigma is related to the key LSS measure Defects Per Million Opportunities (DPMO) that is calculated as follows:

$$DPMO = \frac{Defects}{Opportunities} \times 10^6$$

The DMAIC intervention had been a success, but the improved levels of performance were not sustained. The DMAIC team was reactivated to intervene again.

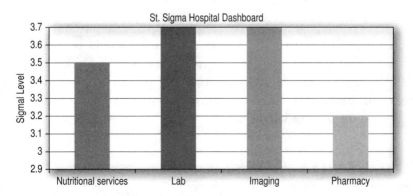

**FIGURE 6-8** St. Sigma Hospital dashboard graphic

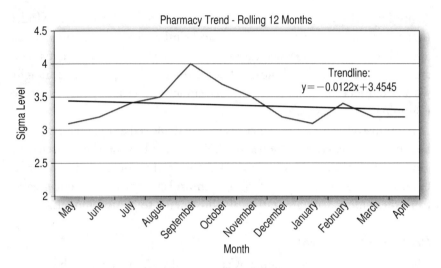

**FIGURE 6-9** St. Sigma Hospital Pharmacy Sigma Level trend

## CONTROL PHASE DELIVERABLES

The key deliverables of the Control Phase are included in a final Control Plan:

- Monitoring plan
- Standardized process flowchart
- Policies and procedures
- Response plan for deterioration in performance
- Transfer of project ownership to process owners

The Control Phase marks the end of the DMAIC intervention and should have demonstrated success. Senior leaders should be included in a session that presents the final project report to stakeholders, and the DMAIC team should be provided with the opportunity to discuss their work and demonstrate specific expertise gained during the project.

Finally, the team should be rewarded. How about a nice game of chess?

## DISCUSSION QUESTIONS

1. What is the purpose of the Control Phase? Why is it the last step in the DMAIC approach?

2. Why does the Control Plan need to include a flowchart? What kinds of flowcharts are typically useful as part of the Control Plan?
3. Describe Deming's System of Profound Knowledge. What does he mean by "drive out fear"?
4. What is the purpose of standardization in quality deployment? Provide an example of a standardization approach in clinical quality improvement.
5. What are the key elements of a training plan?
6. How are the effects of training measured at the personal, business unit, and organizational levels? Provide an example of the application of the Kirkpatrick model from your experience.
7. Describe the elements of a monitoring plan. How are performance targets set?
8. What role does Root Cause Analysis play in the Monitoring Plan?
9. What does the term "poka yoke" mean? Why does the Control Plan need to include this activity?
10. Describe two approaches to poka yoke and give examples from your experience.
11. What is an audit plan? Describe the five phases of the plan.
12. What is the goal of an audit? What types of approaches may be counterproductive during an audit?
13. How are control charts used in the Control Phase?
14. Describe seasonal adjustment. When would seasonal adjustment approaches make sense for analyzing data?
15. Describe clinical risk adjustment. Why is risk adjustment important in data analysis of clinical processes?
16. How is process sigma level used to monitor processes? What are the advantages? What are the disadvantages?

# OTHER RESOURCES

### Checklists

- Pennsylvania Department of Health Transition Health Care Checklist: Accessed April, 2011 at http://www.dsf.health.state.pa.us/health/lib/health/familyhealth/transition_hc_checklistrevised3-07.pdf
- AHRQ checklist for women's preventive health issues and services: Accessed April, 2011 at http://www.ahrq.gov/ppip/healthywom.htm

- Adolescent Autonomy Checklist, Washington Department of Health, Accessed April, 2011 at http://depts.washington.edu/healthtr/Checklists/health_care.htm
- Environmental stewardship checklist for hospitals, Kansas State University, Accessed April 2011 at http://depts.washington.edu/healthtr/Checklists/health_care.htm

# RISK ADJUSTMENT

- American Medical Association Practice Management Center, An introduction to risk assessment and risk adjustment models, Accessed April, 2011 at http://www.ama-assn.org/resources/doc/psa/risk-assessment.pdf.
- Centers for Medicare and Medicaid Services, Risk adjustment, Accessed April, 2011 at https://www.cms.gov/MedicareAdvtgSpecRateStats/06_Risk_adjustment.asp.
- Society of Actuaries, Winkelman R, Mehmud S, A comparative analysis of claims-based tools for health risk assessment, Accessed April, 2011, at http://www.soa.org/files/pdf/risk-assessmentc.pdf.
- Iezzoni L (ed.), *Risk adjustment for measuring healthcare outcomes,* 3rd ed., 2003, Health Administration Press, Chicago.

# REFERENCES

1. W. Edwards Deming Institute. (2011). *The Deming system of profound knowledge.* Retrieved from http://deming.org/index.cfm?content=66.
2. Maslow, A. (1987). *Motivation and personality,* (3rd ed.). New York: Harper & Row Publishers, Inc. Retrieved from http://www.chaight.com/Wk%2015%20E205B%20Maslow%20-%20Human%20Motivation.pdf
3. Field, M.J., & Lohr, K.N. (Eds). (1990). *Clinical practice guidelines: Directions for a new program, Institute of Medicine.* Washington, DC: National Academy Press.
4. Gawande, A.( 2011). *The checklist manifesto: How to get things right.* New York: Picador.
5. Kirkpatrick, D.L., & Kirkpatrick, J.D. (2005). *Transferring learning to behavior: Using the four levels to improve performance.* San Francisco: Berrett-Koehler Publishers, Inc.
6. Grout, J. *Mistake proofing the design of health care processes.* (2007). AHRQ Publication No. 07-0020, May 2007. Retrieved from http://www.ahrq.gov/qual/mistakeproof/mistakeproofing.pdf.

7. Kuzniewicz, M.W., Vasilevskis E.E., Lane, R., Dean, M.L., Trivedi, N.G., Rennie D.J., Clay, T., Kotler, P.L., & Dudley, R.A. Variation in ICU risk adjusted mortality: Impact of methods of assessment and potential confounders. *Chest*, Jun, 133(6), 1319–1327.
8. Richardson, D., Tarnow-Mordi, W.O., & Lee, S.K. (1999). Risk adjustment for quality improvement. *Pediatrics*, 103:1, Supplement January, 255–265.
9. Fry, D.E., Pine, M.B., Jordan, H.S., Hoaglin, D.C., Jones, B., & Meimban, R. (2006). The hazards of using administrative data to measure surgical quality, *American Surgeon*, 72(11), 1031–1037.

# CHAPTER 7

# LSS Case Studies in Health Care

*"Quality means doing it right when no one is looking."*

—Henry Ford

*"The quality of a person's life is in direct proportion to their commitment to excellence, regardless of their chosen field of endeavor."*

—Vince Lombardi

*"Quality is never an accident; it is always the result of intelligent effort."*

—John Ruskin

*"Be willing to make decisions. That's the most important quality in a good leader. Don't fall victim to what I call the ready-aim-aim-aim-aim syndrome. You must be willing to fire."*

—Anonymous

Putting quality into practice is one of the hardest jobs in health care today. No longer can industry leaders say that they must have a quality operation because "we're so busy." A full waiting room or long waiting time do not connote high demand due to quality–they usually indicate an inefficient operation with unneeded variation and higher cost. The world has changed, and highly effective healthcare organizations have changed with it. This chapter is devoted to case studies of projects completed by these organizations, based on reports in the literature and via the Web.

# MIAMI BAPTIST HOSPITAL

**Problem statement:**

The 520-bed hospital in Miami was encountering high levels of inpatient bed utilization and heavy emergency department usage. Senior managers worked with a consultant to use the LSS DMAIC approach to examine and ameliorate the problem.

**Define:**

The hospital and consultant identified two goals: 1) improve the patient discharge process without adding to patient stress or dissatisfaction, and 2) reduce costs and improve overall financial performance.

**Measure: quality tools/approaches:**

The team reviewed process flows and discharge statistics in several areas, using flowchart analysis and evaluating discharge patterns. Additionally, patient data were collected to determine customer satisfaction with these processes.

**Analyze:**

The team discovered that 60% of discharges occurred on the afternoon and evening shifts after 2 p.m., and that the discharge process was creating patient and family dissatisfaction.

**Improve:**

The group divided into five teams to address five different issues:

- Pediatrics
- Triage
- Fast track
- Time to diagnosis
- Time to discharge

The teams applied several change management concepts:

- Engagement of hospitalists to expedite the discharge process
- Improved availability of diagnostic test results
- Emergency department control of the bed overflow unit
- Improvements in the discharge process to expedite patient departure

**Quality metric changes:**
- Discharges prior to 2 p.m. increased from 41% to 80%
- Emergency department hours worked per patient visit decreased by 22%
- Emergency department length of stay decreased by 41%
- Patient-left-without-treatment rates fell from 8% to less than 1%
- Direct admissions to patient floors increased by 181%, reducing the load on the emergency department and decreasing the number of patients in the emergency department waiting for a bed by 37%

**Cost reduction/revenue enhancement:**
- Cost reduction of $4.2 million

**Control:**
- Tracking and intervention systems to identify and remediate lagging performance

**Comments:**

Miami Baptist faced a common problem in hospitals (i.e., the bottleneck), which is an example of Goldratt's Theory of Constraints. In this case, the most significant constraint appeared to relate to the ability to get patients discharged expeditiously and free up beds for admissions from the ED. However, the flow in the ED also presented problems and required interventions to remove barriers to flow. These issues were vetted by teams that focused in five different areas, and the metrics chosen focused on both flow and expense-related concerns. The control program for this intervention was not well described in the literature, but the use of tracking systems with specific interventions for disparities makes the control program effective in dealing with long-term sustainability of the intervention.

**Further information:**

- Miami Baptist Hospital:  http://www.baptisthealth.net
- Caldwell Butler & Associates:  http://www.CaldwellButler.com

# POCONO MEDICAL CENTER (PMC), EAST STROUDSBURG, PA

## Problem statement:

Physicians require laboratory tests at the time of patient rounds, about 7:00 a.m. each morning, to make modifications in patients' care plans.

## Define:

Drawing and processing patients' blood work was not meeting the time constraint of availability by 7:00 a.m. Walter Hays, director of lab services, and Dr. Carmine Cerra, chief of pathology, surveyed the hospital's 160 doctors and found that the CTQ for the medical staff was to have test results available by 7:00 a.m. Further definition of the CTQ indicated that physicians needed critical care patient results by 6:00 a.m. and other patient results by 7:00 a.m. In the laboratory, technicians did not have an effective way to forecast number of blood draws and tests to be done each morning until the middle night, even though orders for morning blood draws were entered throughout the previous day. ICU patients often had scheduled early morning blood draws. Additionally, as phlebotomists drew the blood each morning, they would wait until they had eight to ten samples before taking them to the lab for processing.

## Measure: quality tools/approaches:

Measurement phase involved tracking each tube of blood throughout the process using direct observation by consultants. **A process flowchart** described the process and included time ranges for each step. Four areas emerged as constraints:

- Sample collection
- Sample delivery to the lab
- Initial processing of sample in lab
- Test execution

## Analyze:

The data were analyzed using several statistical tools:

- Time series plots
- Control charts
- Stratified frequency plots
- Hypothesis tests (e.g., ANOVA)
- Multiple regression
- Pareto charts
- Binary logistic regression

The analyses revealed that the largest bottleneck was the practice of collecting ten to fifteen samples before returning the batch of samples to the lab for processing. Not only was the wait time substantial, the batch created a "bump" in the process. Analysis of the data indicated that every 7.5 minutes a phlebotomist could draw between one and four tubes of blood.

## Improve:

A laboratory person was designated to retrieve samples from the patient care unit every 15 minutes during the peak time in the morning. Phlebotomists indicate their current location with a flasher light outside the room in which they are currently drawing blood so that the lab runner can find them easily.

## Quality metric changes:

| | | Time | % results delivered on time |
|---|---|---|---|
| Standard patient units | Before intervention | 7 a.m. | 68% |
| | After intervention | 7 a.m. | 98% |
| | | Time | % results delivered on time |
| ICU/CCU/PCU | 6 a.m. | Before intervention | 18% |
| | | After intervention | 92% |
| | 7 a.m. | Before intervention | 81% |
| | | After intervention | 100% |

**Cost reduction/revenue enhancement:**

- Because the flow improved so dramatically, the lab did not require an increase in staff to implement the new process.
- Improved lab delivery times also contributed to a reduced length of stay.

**Control:**

- The intervention was completed in six weeks.
- Buy in from the medical staff improved the rate of progress, and the resulting improvement in physician satisfaction with result delivery times was remarkable.
- The process is monitored closely, and the staff intervenes if the timeliness metric falls below 95% or if variance exceeds 10%; however, all late test are reviewed for improvement.

**Comments:**

This case is a good example of how a seemingly minor issue, the ability of phlebotomists to get blood samples to the lab expeditiously, has downstream repercussions. Physicians require lab and imaging data during rounds that allow them to make decisions about a patient's care over the next few hours, and lacking that data, requests for interventions can be delayed, with increased chance for errors as treatments might be delayed or omitted. Additionally, many healthcare systems measure physician satisfaction as a way to ensure that the organization is meeting the needs of the medical staff so that they will continue to use the facility and services for their patients. This project team performed the appropriate root cause analysis to track the underlying process nonconformities, and the analysis revealed significant opportunities for improvement. Importantly, the team found interventions, such as the "lab runners," to ameliorate these problems inexpensively and expeditiously. Physician buy-in to the solution was important, but the results (i.e., greater availability of on time lab tests) likely had a substantial effect on medical staff support. Finally, the Control Phase had effective metrics and well-defined interventions for ensuring long-term success of the project.

**Further information:**

Pocono Medical Center:               http://www.poconohealthsystem.org
Pocono Medical Center laboratory:  http://www.pmclab.org

# NEBRASKA MEDICAL CENTER PEGGY D. COWDERY PATIENT CARE CENTER

**Problem statement:**

Physicians' orders received from multiple possible sources were incomplete and could be lost, jeopardizing patient safety.

**Define:**

The Nebraska Medical Center's Peggy D. Cowdery Patient Care Center (CPCC), the organization's 26-bed cancer treatment facility, had multiple potential intake mechanisms for physician orders. The Center's 260 physicians could send orders from one of the 15 Nebraska Medical Center locations, or send them by phone or fax. Incomplete orders were difficult to track back to their source for completion, orders could be misplaced, or multiple copies of orders could exist, all of which can delay care and invariably lead to staff and patient dissatisfaction. Not only were patients and staff frustrated, but the risk to patient safety was also extant in the unorganized approach to order entry and execution. An eight-member team was assembled from within and outside the CPCC staff, and they quickly identified the major issues:

- Multiple entry points for physician orders
- All eight of the CPCC's clerical staff entered orders
- The clerk responsible for fielding future orders also was tasked with answering phones and running errands throughout the hospital.
- Storage cabinets for the telephone and fax orders were at least 100 feet from the order entry clerk's desk.
- Patients with infrequent appointments often had their orders placed in the drawer without appropriate filing.
- Lack of filing guidelines allowed orders to be placed in a filing cabinet, at order drop-off points, or in a nurse's chart.

**Measure: quality tools/approaches:**

The team developed metrics for each of the key process steps that were suspected to be flawed. Baseline measurements were made for each of the measures over a two-day period.

## Analyze:

As the team analyzed the data, they determined that no specific factor could be attributed as the cause of the inconsistent performance. Instead, multiple points in the process lacked sufficient rigor to ensure a favorable outcome. These points constituted the "critical-x" values that the team targeted for improvement.

## Improve:

Rather than try to repair the dysfunctional process with multiple opportunities for improvement, the team created "Order Central" using lean concepts of putting workers with parallel or intersecting workflows close together to improve communications and reduce transport time for shared materials and data. "Order Central" staffing consisted of two clerical staff members and a triage nurse, and they were relocated to the check-in/check-out area, where they engaged in implementing a number of process changes:

- Patient charts were placed in a location adjacent to Order Central
- The "catch-all" drawer, where many orders were misplaced, was no longer used
- Order acceptance points were reduced from fifteen to three: 1) at the check-out desk, 2) a bin near Order Central for nonurgent orders, and 3) a bin above the Order Central clerk's workstation for orders requiring immediate attention
- Order Central phones were programmed to limit incoming calls to a manageable number
- Training sessions increased visibility of the issue of incomplete orders
- Each practitioner who could enter patient orders (case managers, physicians, and midlevel practitioners) were provided with individual performance reports on completeness of orders
- The form that practitioners used for entering and submitting orders was simplified

## Quality metric changes:

The team measured order completeness failure and order availability failure rates for a six-month period following the changes with the following results:

| Metric | Baseline | Month | | | | | |
|---|---|---|---|---|---|---|---|
| | | 1 | 2 | 3 | 4 | 5 | 6 |
| Orders incomplete | 29% | 7% | 9% | 8% | 4% | 7% | 3% |
| Orders not available | 59% | 21% | 21% | 8% | 8% | 9% | 0.08% |

In addition to the operational metric improvements, the organization realized significant improvements in the NRC-Picker patient satisfaction survey positive responses, with the overall rating showing a rise from the 90th percentile to the 100th percentile.

### Cost reduction/revenue enhancement:

Cost data were not presented in the report, but gains in productivity can be anticipated from elimination of nonvalue-added work to find missing results and time spent redoing order sets for patients whose orders are missing. Additionally, gains in patient safety may also be anticipated from the availability and accuracy of patient orders. All of these results were achieved at relatively little cost (i.e., moving desks and electronic equipment to the new location).

### Control:

The team uses the metrics developed during the Analyze Phase to monitor the new process to ensure that the current state of control is maintained.

### Comments:

Ambulatory centers with multiple points of contact are prone to errors, and this oncology center had so many potential entry points for physician orders that many order sets were incomplete or contained errors that had implications for patient safety. Because of the level of dysfunction of the current process, the team decided to completely revise the entire process. The redesign not only changed the process flow, but also the location of the process team. Using the lean principle of one-piece flow, the people who were involved in managing incoming orders were placed in a pod, centrally located, and passage of the information was streamlined to reduce the number of touches. The team also introduced a flow-limiting step by limiting incoming call rates, ensuring that the order takers had sufficient time to receive complete order sets. Although this approach adds a constraint to the process flow, the bottleneck is important to reduce errors and improve quality. Another approach to this problem might entail adding more staff to manage a higher volume of calls, but this method might add an inordinate amount of cost to the process, and a cost benefit analysis will help determine the best way to create value in these situations.

One important point to note in this case is the elimination of the "catch-all" drawer, which was instrumental in perpetuating the errors in the process. Analysis of the process flow generally identifies these nonconformities so that the team can remove the source of error. Additionally, providing order writers with their error rates for order completion through feedback reports is another effective control strategy that can be an important factor in reducing the human source of error.

Nearly all Six Sigma projects attempt to quantify the economic benefits of the project. In this case, the financial results were not provided, but cost data could be collected for a number of factors. For example, personnel time wasted during searches for incomplete orders could be collected and totaled to determine the cost of the unproductive time. Other possible financial metrics could be attributed to the risk of malpractice losses if a patient is injured or mistreated because of the lack of orders, or at the very least the reduced number of staff members required to support the new process. Since most of these types of projects have substantial cost savings associated with removal of waste or risk, the use of financial metrics as a method of demonstrating the value of the project makes sense.

**Further information:**

- Nebraska Medical Center :     http://www.nebraskamed.com

# RADIA, INC.

**Project name:**

On-time MRI scans

**Problem statement:**

Radia, Inc. is a vascular surgery and radiology practice in the Pacific Northwest. After the MRI equipment at the Evergreen Radia Imaging Center was upgraded, the number of scans performed per technologist per day dropped to 20% below the best-performing Radia outpatient center and 8% below the industry benchmark.

## Define:

The site medical director and operations director determined that 53% of patients who had scans on the new equipment had start times for the procedure that was more than 5 minutes after the scheduled start time, and so they decided to commission an improvement team to investigate and reach a target of 60% on time procedure starts, which would also increase the number of scans performed with a concomitant rise of $200,000 annual revenue. During this phase, the team of MRI technologists mapped the process of care, and several potential bottlenecks were identified, such as:

- As the MRI tech was monitoring the computer for the arrival of the next patient, the tech was often diverted by other tasks and missed the patient's arrival.
- As patients waited for the procedure, they completed forms to identify risk factors for the MRI study, like an implanted pacemaker, or a cochlear implant. Even if the patient completed the forms in a timely manner, they were often not called for the procedure until after the scheduled start time if the tech did not become aware of the safety issue until just prior to the scan. The team interviewed patients to discern the Voice of the Customer (VOC) and learned that less than 5 minutes between the scheduled and actual procedure start time would be considered "exceptional performance."

## Measure: quality tools/approaches:

The team agreed on a key metric of "appointment to scan time," defined as the time interval between a patient's scheduled appointment time and the time that a scan begins. A SIPOC diagram was constructed to help understand the inputs and outputs for each phase of the process, and the team determined that 79% of the x-variables were controllable. The customer CTQs obtained from the VOC were used to prioritize the input variables and reduce the list to 18 key process inputs. Team members were trained in data collection, and cycle time data was collected during routine operations using standardized forms that had been calibrated by staff and separate observers to ensure accurate data collection. From these data, the team ascertained:

- Mean appointment-to-scan time was 7.5 minutes with a median of 3 minutes

- Range was −32 minutes to +120 minutes
- The scheduled appointment duration often did not match the actual scan time (i.e., the time allotted for the scan was not the same as the time it took to complete the scan).
- A control chart demonstrated that the scanning processes had no special causes (i.e., that the variation was exclusively common cause).

The team conducted an FMEA to identify problems that could occur in the process and used that information to anticipate potential problems.

## Analyze:

The team viewed the data in a number of ways, such as a Pareto chart to categorize types of problems and performed a second FMEA to identify problems that actually occurred, resulting in immediate development and deployment of a new patient safety form to better capture issues in the patient's history that could complicate the scan. The analysis continued with statistical tests (Fisher's Exact test) to demonstrate that the techs were performing similarly, and a two-sample t-test to demonstrate that the new safety form took significantly less time for the patient to complete. Another two-sample t-test demonstrated that problems such as patients arriving late or having claustrophobia did not significantly add to the delay in starting the scan. A classic bar chart was used to show that the median scan time of 26 minutes contributed substantially to patient flow through the MRI facility. The result of these analyses indicated that the patient safety form was the most significant critical x for the Improve Phase.

## Improve:

The two improvement opportunities that the analysis identified for intervention are 1) the check-in process and completion of forms and 2) scan prep during which the tech interviews the patient and deals with the patient's safety issues prior to initiating the scan. The improvement plan thus included:

- Patient interview during the check-in process at the time of the patient's arrival at the clinic conducted by a patient service representative—used to identify patient safety issues or contraindications to the scan.

- Full factorial design of experiments (DOE) that tested the revised safety form and the new check-in process. The DOE required 52 runs, half of which were done with patients and half with staff.

Review of these improvements indicated that the revised check-in process with the patient interview had a greater impact on time to procedure than did the new patient safety form, since the form still required tech time to review and follow up on any ambiguities. The interview process effectively reduced the time to identify a patient safety issue from a mean of 15.9 minutes to less than 1 minute.

Informal ways of dealing with patient safety issues were shared during brainstorming sessions in the Analyze Phase and applied less rigorously during the Improve Phase, and the effects of these changes were not quantified. Additional changes in work patterns were tested in the Improve Phase, and the resulting conclusions included:

- The revised safety-screening form and interview process at the time of the patient's arrival was demonstrated to be efficacious and were adopted.
- The process would add the requirement to notify techs at the time of the patient's arrival and the results of the safety interview.
- One tech is dedicated to preparing patients for the scanner to eliminate the extra time needed for preparation.
- Have one technologist serve as a lead tech to coordinate flow.
- Use new procedures developed by the radiologist for patients with claustrophobia or who move during the test.
- Document new standardized operating procedures.
- Standardize all appointments to 30 minute time allotments.

**Quality metric changes:**

| Intervention | Baseline | Post-intervention |
|---|---|---|
| Form | 10.5 min | 5.5 min |
| Check-in interview | 15.9 min | 1 min |
| All interventions | 7.5 min | −1.1 min |

**Cost reduction/revenue enhancement:**
- The clinic was able to add seven additional scans per weekday
- Annual revenue projections increased by $1.4 million

**Control:**

The monitoring program uses a p-chart to monitor process stability. The new goal that was set by the clinic is 75% of on-time scans, and performance for that metric is monitored by a bar chart that is shared with the staff. The clinic has met that new goal in four out of six months, and the team is working to improve performance by cross training and improving orientation of part time and substitute techs who cover the clinic during staff vacations. At the time of the report, the clinic was operating at 21% over the expected number of scans.

**Comments:**

One of the primary purposes of lean is to remove nonvalue-added (NVA) work from a process, and this case is a good example of detecting and eliminating the NVA work. The SIPOC diagram not only helped determine process flow, but it also helped define which input variables could be altered to improve the process. Critical x-values were then identified using Six Sigma tools like Pareto analysis and FMEA, which provided further data for tests of statistical significance that narrowed the critical x-values to the important few that could be affected by an intervention. As critical x-values were pared, the team found a clear opportunity for intervention in the process that patients followed on intake that involved completion of a safety form. The team conducted a full factorial DOE, that consisted of 52 runs, which is often difficult to implement because of cost or time, but from those experiments the team identified multiple changes to the process that ultimately proved effective in reducing both the throughput metrics, but also increasing the projected revenue because of the ability to handle higher volumes of patients in the new process.

The control process is particularly remarkable, since it uses a control chart to monitor stability. Not only were control limits calculated but specification limits were also set, and through cross training and better orientation of part time techs greater compliance with the new process was achieved.

**Further information:**

Radia, Inc.:    http://www.radiax.com

# PROVIDENCE ST. JOSEPH MEDICAL CENTER (PSJMC), BURBANK, CA

**Project name:**

Surgical infection prevention

**Problem statement:**

PSJMC is a nonprofit 448-bed acute care hospital in Burbank with an active surgery program (over 4500 procedures annually). As part of their patient safety and quality program, PSJMC participates in the Center of Medicare and Medicaid Services (CMS) Surgical Care Improvement Program (SCIP) and collects data for evaluating standardized measures for that program.[1] One metric in particular, SCIP 3 (discontinuation of antibiotic prophylaxis within 24 hours post-op), had remained consistently low at 36%, which was the hospital's worst performance on any national quality measure. The Six Sigma project was directed at improving performance on that measure.

**Define:**

PSJMC's objective is to be at the 90th percentile for all national quality measures, which for the SCIP 3 metric was 95% compliance with recommendations for discontinuation of antibiotics within 24 hours after surgery. Thus, the goal of the project is to improve performance on the SCIP 3 metric from 36% compliance to at least 95% compliance. The Six Sigma team was assembled from stakeholders from all affected clinical areas, and both day and night shifts, including physicians. The team gathered data from a number of sources:

- Nursing staff focus groups
- Physician surveys
- Physician order sets
- Antibiotic prophylaxis drug order data
- Flowchart of the antibiotic prophylaxis process

The team carefully limited the scope of the project to avoid project creep and make the goal unachievable.

The team determined that the poor performance on the SCIP 3 measure was due to several factors:

- Lack of understanding of the requirements of the SCIP 3 metric (i.e., the evidence-based recommendation for discontinuation of antibiotics in certain patients at 24 hours post-operatively)
- Resistance to changing current practices, often specialty specific
- Poor communication and collaboration between pharmacy, operating room, and nursing units
- Lack of a SCIP 3 operational procedure
- No oversight of SCIP 3 compliance on weekends
- No standard medical staff order sets
- Lack of a process to identify patients who qualified for SCIP 3 measurement

**Measure: quality tools/approaches:**

The team used the flowchart and patient chart data to analyze each step in the antibiotic prophylaxis process. Measures included:

- Type and complexity of the surgery
- Definition of surgery end time
- Order set used
- Ordering physician
- Type, dosage, frequency of antibiotics
- Time of last dose of antibiotic
- For antibiotics administered after the 24-hour cutoff, reason for lack of compliance

Staff members involved in collecting chart data were trained in the specific requirements for this study, but obtaining timely data was still difficult because of the time required and complexity for abstracting data from the paper charts by the quality department staff. Additionally, accuracy and consistency of data obtained via this type of chart review is always questionable. The data collected provided several key measures:

| Measure | Baseline performance |
|---|---|
| Average stop time of antibiotic therapy post-op | 39 hours |
| Compliance with SCIP 3 guidelines | 25% |

| Measure | Baseline performance |
|---|---|
| Presence of standardized SCIP 3 process on nursing units | No |
| Pharmacy involvement in discontinuation process | No |

**Analyze:**

Using process map reviews and root cause analysis, the team analyzed the data using statistical techniques like time series charts and chi-square tests to determine rates of compliance with the discontinuation guidelines and then to further segment the data in a number of ways (e.g., by specialty) to prioritize intervention needs. The team found that the highest rates of noncompliance occurred among orthopedic and colorectal surgeons, who performed 50% of the surgical procedures on SCIP 3 eligible patients. The team conducted interviews with each noncompliant doctor after thoroughly reviewing all of the surgeon's potential SCIP 3 patients and then explained to the surgeon the issues of noncompliance found in the charts based on the standard definitions. In spite of the evidence regarding the appropriateness of the SCIP 3 discontinuation criteria, some surgeons, primarily orthopedists, resisted change to their routine practices. The analyses confirmed the findings from the Define Phase regarding barriers to compliance with the guideline.

**Improve:**

The team met with key stakeholders to explain the data and then brainstormed approaches to removing the barriers to good care. The team came up with the following potential solutions:

- Work with physicians to create new or revised SCIP 3 compliant order sets
- Collection and review of patient data sheets at each transition to a new clinical unit to allow the nurse manager to understand daily compliance with SCIP 3 criteria
- Automation of discontinuation orders at the pharmacy at 24 hours post-operatively approved by the Medical Executive Committee
- Screen patients in the operating room to identify those who meet SCIP 3 criteria and fax that information to short-stay, pharmacy, and nursing units
- Put orange stickers on patient charts to alert others to the SICP 3 patients

The team produced a new flowchart of the revised SCIP 3 process for piloting on two nursing units with large numbers of SCIP 3 patients. The pilot test identified a number of other issues (e.g., that the quality team and clinical units also needed to receive the list of SCIP 3 patients). After appropriate revisions based on pilot test findings, the new process was implemented in other units and the ICU.

The team concentrated throughout the Improve Phase on roles and responsibilities of each stakeholder, as well as the overarching goal. Physician champions helped gain physician adoption of the new approach, and improvement team members interacted with stakeholders frequently throughout this phase.

### Quality metric changes:

The key metric for the project, SCIP 3 compliance, demonstrated a favorable outcome as the new process was implemented, rising from a month-to-month range of 20–60% to a month-to-month range of 82–100% compliance after the intervention was completely deployed. This new level of performance was more consistently at the 90th percentile target set by PSJMC for this project.

Additionally, nursing and pharmacy staff members now perceive an increased focus on quality of care and improved working relationships with all providers involved in each patient's care.

### Cost reduction/revenue enhancement:

Cost savings from the project are estimated at $35,000 annually.

### Control:

The team set up a number of monitoring processes to ensure that the process remained in control, including:

- Automating the antibiotic discontinuation order at the pharmacy
- Quality management specialist rounds daily on hospital units to check list of SCIP 3 patients against actual orders and treatments
- Medical staff oversight by Surgical Quality Improvement Council to deal with noncompliant physicians

Additionally, the approach was deployed to other hospitals in the parent organization with similar results.

## Comments:

CMS' SCIP measures have set the standard for surgical care in the past few years, and combined with the American College of Surgeons (ACS) Nora Institute for Surgical Patient Safety (http://www.surgicalpatientsafety. facs.org/index.html), the measures and resulting improvement projects should help ensure advances in error reduction and safety in the operative theater. SCIP 3 is a metric that was designed to ensure that antibiotic prophylaxis administered just prior to surgery is then stopped 24 hours after surgery in certain procedures to reduce the growing problem of bacterial resistance to antibiotics. Surgeons are cautious about postoperative infections, and many were trained years ago when continuation of antibiotic prophylaxis beyond 24-hours post-op was commonplace. However, more recent evidence[2] indicates that continuation of prophylaxis past 24 hours does not improve patient outcomes for most surgical procedures, and overuse of antibiotics can lead to development of "superbugs" that are resistant to multiple antibiotics and therefore difficult or impossible to treat. As indicated in the reference, antibiotic discontinuation is a hard habit to break, and many hospitals are challenged with the same issues as PSJMC.

During the Define Phase, the team discovered that resistance among the surgeons was only one of many problems, the most significant of which was the lack of any formalized process to implement the standard of antibiotic prophylaxis timing and in many cases a lack of understanding of the recommendation. The Analyze Phase was particularly telling, with the data showing that 50% of patients in the SCIP 3 measurement set had colorectal or orthopedic procedures, and those two surgical specialties were particularly resistant to adhering to the new standards. This situation presents a special challenge, so the team met individually with noncompliant physicians to explain the evidence for the revised practice and achieved some gains with these specialists.

The team then proceeded to set up a process that institutionalized the process through routine order sets and automatic discontinuation orders for prophylactic antibiotics. All of these changes netted significant improvements in performance on SCIP 3, from 20–60% month-to-month compliance to 80–100% compliance after the intervention, which has persisted after several cycles. Since the process sigma was not reported, the degree of improvement in process capability was not explicit.

This project demonstrates one of the major issues that clinical improvement programs face in every setting (i.e., physician preference and a reliance on experience rather than on evidence-based medicine [EBM]). Since physicians hold the "power of the pen" and influence or direct the vast majority of healthcare services and expenditures, numerous approaches have been mounted to deal with this influence, such as the creation of clinical practice guidelines (CPGs) based on EBM, various utilization management interventions, attempts to incentivize physicians for complying with specific recommendations, and development of penalties for noncompliance. In this case, the team used another of the common approaches (i.e., direct discussions with physicians) usually conducted by a "physician champion" who can relate to the practitioner and counter objections with sound experimentally-based evidence and the champion's own clinical experience. This approach appears to have been effective, since improvement in compliance doubled after the interventions. The relative contribution of this approach versus the other interventions was not apparently measured, but physician engagement in a clinical improvement project is nearly always a crucial step to ensure success.

Finally, the cost savings of $35,000 was likely the direct-cost savings from avoiding excessive use of medications. On the other hand, the costs associated with treatment of patient infections due to resistant bacterial agents are immense, and the treatments are often unsuccessful leading to patient death. Thus, although these costs are difficult to quantify, the reality of these types of infections and the benefits of avoiding them should at least be recognized as a positive benefit of the intervention.

**Further information:**

- PSJMC website:   http://www2.providence.org/saintjoseph/Pages/default.aspx

# NORTH SHORE-LONG ISLAND JEWISH HEALTH SYSTEM, NEW YORK CITY

**Project name:**

CT scan throughput improvement

## Problem statement:

North Shore-Long Island Jewish (NSLIJ) Health System faced an issue with radiology throughput creating satisfaction issues with patients and providers. The organization focused its efforts on two CT scanners to optimize flow through these resources.

## Define:

Turnaround times (TAT) for CT scans were below the expectations of key customers like physicians, case management nurses, and hospital leadership. The organization measured the VOC of these stakeholders and the expected time for completion of the test was 16 hours, but the average TAT for these procedures was 20.7 hours with a range of 8 to 34 hours. NSLIJ formed a LSS team consisting of physician, technical, managerial, transport, and clerical staff from the radiology department and LSS staff from the health system's Center of Learning and Innovation. The team was charged with improving average daily patient throughput to national best-in-class benchmarks by increasing patient volume by 20% during regular business hours (Monday–Friday from 8:00 a.m. to midnight), which translated into increasing patient volume from 45 patients per day to 54 patients per day.

Baseline performance data were collected, including VOC data and current volumes of patients. From these inquiries, the team found the following:

- CT techs answered up to 75 calls per day regarding scheduling questions, which reduced their availability to perform scans
- The work environment was unorganized and lacked a workspace for the lead technologist
- CT techs opined that preparation and delivery of oral contrast media were not efficient
- Pretransport processes and transporter availability were not optimal

The team planned a Kaizen event to attack the problem. Black Belts prepared a number of the tools for the Kaizen, such as scope definition, collection of baseline data, and creation of a charter. The chair of the radiology department for the NSLIJ Health System was the executive sponsor of the project. The event lasted four days and implementation began immediately after the event.

## Measure:

The first day of the event started with the Measure Phase, which included a validation stage to ensure that the measurement systems designed by the Black Belts accurately collected and computed measures. The team defined a TAT defect as any scan that took more than 16 hours from the time the CT was ordered until the test is performed, and using that definition the process sigma was computed to be 1.7s (398,358 DPMO). The Kaizen team created a value stream map of the CT ordering and completion process and labeled each step with one of three categories:

- **Value added (VA)**–essential to provide the service to the customer
- **Business nonvalue added (BNVA)**–required for business purposes, but no additional value for the customer
- **Nonvalue added (NVA)**–no business or customer value

The team looked for the seven deadly wastes (muda) using the value stream map:

- Transportation
- Inventory
- Wasted motion
- Waiting
- Overproduction
- Overprocessing
- Defects and rework

Key metrics included the number of patients scanned and reasons for cancellation. Additionally, CT techs and transporters wore pedometers to determine how many steps each worker took each day, which provided interesting data:

- CT techs traveled 6,480 feet each day to the printer devoted to CT scan requisitions because the printer was down a hall away from the scanners; this NVA activity amounted to 324 miles per year of movement that did not add value to the process.
- Transporters averaged 432 feet per day moving back and forth to the transport notification printer, adding 21.6 miles of NVA movement per year.

**Analyze:**

Vital x-values were identified using an Ishikawa cause-and-effect diagram that was organized into three major categories: workspace, workflow, and scheduling. The cluttered workplace was ideal for a 5S intervention, and that effort freed up space for the lead technologist who was responsible for helping expedite patient flow, but other improvements were also possible, including another computer workstation and file storage shelves.

The Kaizen team then examined workflow using the value stream map and spaghetti diagrams, and multiple sources of NVA were found, such as the wasted motion data discovered by the pedometer measurements. The team also turned attention to scheduling issues, and the problem with CT techs managing scheduling phone calls in addition to their duties to perform scans was further analyzed to reveal that the root cause was the manual scheduling process, which made information about patient appointment times poorly available. The lack of general availability of the schedule also led to delays when the patient's nurse was unaware that a study had been scheduled.

**Improve:**

The third day of the Kaizen event was devoted to developing and testing improvements based on the analysis conducted on day two, and several potential solutions arose:

- Wasted motion (the many miles walking to the printers)—one printer was used for both scan requests and transport requests located closer to the scanning room that eliminated about 300 miles per year per technician in wasted motion. The new location and consolidation of scan and transport requests promoted better communication between techs and transporters.
- Allocation of a transporter to the CT department, rather than using transporters from the general transporter pool.
- Reorganization of the reception area included addition of a refrigerator in which contrast media may be stored for distribution to patients by the receptionist.
- Oral contrast preparation was completed by techs on the evening shift, eliminating the task from intruding on tech time during peak volume times.

- Scheduling was automated using Excel®, with schedules faxed to each patient care unit, as well as being available through Microsoft Outlook® throughout the hospital. The availability of the schedule via the computer system reduced the number of calls, as well as the number of cancellations due to improper patient preparation or unavailability.
- As a patient scan is being completed, the next patient on the schedule is brought to the department, rather than waiting for the scheduled time.
- Changes in scheduling rules to eliminate outpatient scans on Mondays to better accommodate the backlog that occurs on weekends. That change led to both increased numbers of inpatients on Mondays (10 more exams), but also increased numbers of patients scanned on the other days of the weeks.
- Designation of one CT scanner for complex procedures and the second for routine, high volume scans.
- Development of a WWW (who, what, when) accountability framework for assigning tasks from the Kaizen event to individual team members.

## Quality metric improvement:

| Measure | Baseline | After Improve Phase |
|---|---|---|
| TAT | 20.7 hours | 11.6 hours |
| Inpatient procedures | | +200 |
| Outpatient procedures | | +60 |
| Patients scanned per day | 45 | 51 |
| Process sigma | 1.7σ | 2.6σ |
| Cancellations due to improper preparation | 30.6% | 22.7% |

## Cost/financial management improvement:
Annual revenue from CT scans increased by $375,000.

## Control:

The fourth day focused on piloting the processes, refining the interventions, and creating a Control Plan. The pilot tests demonstrated an immediate 33% improvement in throughput, and anecdotal feedback indicated that the nursing staff appreciated access to the automated schedule.

Individual-X Moving Range (IXMR) charts were developed to track daily patient volume, and process capability charts were created to track TAT. Results were dramatic, with the performance indicators used to track the process achieving the improved levels in the table within thirty days.

## Comments:

Throughput is a classical lean process management problem, and TAT is the most characteristic measure for these types of projects. Once the flowchart was constructed, dividing the work into three categories (VA, BNVA, NVA) helped the team best decide where to intervene for improvements. Using the seven deadly wastes (muda) of lean, the team was able to find points in the process where significant time was wasted and then focus on specific process changes to eliminate those activities. In many lean-focused projects, simple solutions are often quickly identified (e.g., moving a printer down the hall to eliminate extra steps to retrieve reports or consolidating reports on one printer) to not only reduce overhead, but also to encourage discourse between two different workforce groups.

Another important feature of this case was the use of a Kaizen event to focus the team on the process and expedite interventions. As shown by the Kaizen in this situation, the team can get months' worth of work done in a relatively short time (four days in this case), including prototyping an intervention to determine results, so that the culmination of the event is a set of functioning interventions and a Control Phase plan that will sustain the gains. Another feature of the Kaizen event that should be emphasized is the quantification of worker transit time using pedometers. The revelation that CT techs were walking over 300 miles each year just retrieving reports from the printer indicated not just the existence of wasted motion, but an actual number indicating the degree of NBVA work. Additionally, use of the process sigma level helped demonstrate the overall improvement in the process resulting from the interventions. The team also leveraged existing technology (Microsoft Outlook) to share data, rather than create or purchase a new system to do the same task.

The Control Phase maintained the team's scientific approach by implementing an IX-MR chart to monitor process performance, and just as importantly, the team measured the addition to revenue ($375,000) caused by the improved process flow. In short, this project nicely demonstrated the symbiosis of the Lean and Six Sigma approaches and provides a good example of why these two separately developed improvement systems have coalesced so well in the healthcare industry.

**More information:**

- North Shore-Long Island Jewish website: http://www.northshorelij .com

**Additional resources:**

**Internet sources of case studies**

| Sponsor | Site |
|---|---|
| BMGI | http://www.bmgi.com/browse/case-studies/results |
| Healthcare Performance Partners | http://leanhealthcareperformance.com/leancasestudies.php |
| iSixSigma | http://www.isixsigma.com |
| Scribd | http://www.scribd.com/tag/lean%20healthcare?l=1 |

**Books**

Arthur, J. *Lean Six Sigma for hospitals: Simple steps to fast affordable, and flawless healthcare.* (2011). Columbus, OH: McGraw Hill.

Caldwell, C., Brexler, J., & Gillem, T. (2005). *Lean-Six Sigma for healthcare: A senior leader guide to improving cost and throughput.* Milwaukee, WI: ASQ Quality Press.

Trusko, B.E., Pexton, C., Harrington, H.J., & Gupta, P. (2007). *Improving healthcare quality and cost with Six Sigma.* Upper Saddle River, NJ: Financial Times Press.

# DISCUSSION QUESTIONS

1. For any of the case studies, how was DMAIC applied to solve a specific problem? What was the advantage of using DMAIC?
2. For any of the case studies, what LSS tools were used and why were they selected? Does it appear that the tools produced desired results?
3. Describe the use of TAT for the NSLIJ case study. Why was the metric selected?

4. For many of these case studies, a process sigma was not calculated. How could a process sigma have helped each team in achieving improvement goals?

5. The PSJMC case study demonstrated the need for including specific stakeholders in the improvement process. Which stakeholders were most important in that case? Why?

6. What lean principles did Nebraska Medical Center use in its process transformation? How were those principles applied?

7. How did Goldratt's Theory of Constraints (TOC) apply to Miami Baptist's efforts to improve patient flow? How did the TOC apply to the "Order Central" solution in the Nebraska Medical Center case? Describe the difference.

## REFERENCES

1. Quality Net. Surgical care improvement program (SCIP). Retrieved from http://www.qualitynet.org/dcs/ContentServer?level3=Measures&c=MQParents&pagename=Medqic/Measure/MeasuresHome&cid=1137346750659&parentName=TopicCat.

2. Bratzler, D.W., Houck, P.M., Richards, C., Steele, L., Dellinger, E.P., Fry, D.E., Wright C., Ma, A., Carr, K., & Red, L. (2005). Use of antimicrobial prophylaxis for major surgery, baseline results from the National Surgical Infection Prevention Project. *Archives of Surgery*, 140, 174-182

# CHAPTER 8

# DMAIC in an Era of Reform

*"In 2008, about 750,000 bankruptcies were filed. About 70 percent of those bankruptcies were filed because of healthcare costs. Eighty percent of the people who filed for bankruptcy because of healthcare costs had health insurance. America is the only country in the world where if you get sick or hurt, you're going to have file for bankruptcy."*

—Senate Majority Leader Harry Reid

*"Everybody here understands the desperation that people feel when they're sick. And I think everybody here is profoundly sympathetic and wants to make sure that we have a system that works for all Americans."*

—President Barack Obama

## TRENDS IN HEALTHCARE REFORM

Many of us who have been involved in the quality movement in the healthcare industry feel that our time has come. The Patient Protection and Affordable Care Act (PPACA) of 2010 promises to sweep through the healthcare delivery system in the United States and enhance infrastructure by increasing payment system reliance on measurement and quality of care. The new incentives will no longer require high volume to optimize income, but rather focus on the quality of services provided, patient satisfaction, and reduction in the level of inappropriate costs. PPACA proposes several "new" types of payment programs, but in many ways these approaches repackage historical methods with a new quality-focused nuance that will force healthcare providers to measure processes and outcomes of care to be able to survive in the future. The new quality emphasis will have a profound effect on the practice of medicine, since it will require objective reporting of metrics to nearly all payers. Ten important trends will foster the infrastructure and processes necessary to achieve this level of accountability:

- **Value-based purchasing**–a key component of PPACA is the concept of value-based purchasing (VBP), which considers both cost and quality of care using the value proposition that the value of a service or product is directly related to quality and inversely related to cost. Congress has made the concept of value central to the healthcare system of the future, and that tenet mandates much of the remainder of the provisions of the law. For example, under the mantra of "can't manage what isn't measured," a number of features of the bill and other laws passed recently emphasize the collection and analysis of clinical data to determine the cost and quality of care being delivered. Payers other than CMS have also begun requiring more clinical data to perform these value analyses, as their customers (businesses that buy their health insurance products) are becoming increasingly interested in ensuring that their scarce funds are well invested in the health of their workforce.
- **Meaningful use**–automation of clinical recordkeeping systems became the focus of a program launched by the federal government in 2009 through the Health Information Technology for Economic and Clinical Health (HITECH) Act. Meaningful Use criteria were established for physician use of electronic medical record (EMR) systems, and financial incentives were provided for those physicians who adopted the technology. The goal of this initiative was to get more physicians to put clinical information into a format that could be analyzed without costly and tedious paper chart reviews, thus allowing more effective review of practice patterns for quality.

- **ICD-10 coding**–the healthcare industry has used the ICD-9-CM coding system for clinical diagnoses and some procedural reporting for several decades, and as the knowledge base in medicine has grown, so too has the number and level of detail of diagnoses and procedures, such that the ICD-9-CM coding system is no longer adequate to capture sufficient detail for medical reporting. Computers can analyze coded data much more easily than text, and so coded data provide the greatest ability for the types of population health analyses that will be needed to ensure high quality, low cost care. CMS has determined that provider claims submitted for payment must use the more granular ICD-10 codes by October 2013. This coding system has been used throughout the world since the 1980s, but the United States healthcare system has been slow to change. The now firm deadline of October, 2013 ensures that provider and payer billing systems will have the capacity to handle these codes, so analysts and epidemiologists will soon have much more detail for the assessments needed to improve quality and lower cost.
- **Physicians' Quality Reporting Initiative (PQRI)**–this program started in 2006 as a method of getting physicians accustomed to reporting quality data to the Centers for Medicare and Medicaid Services (CMS), as well as validating reporting and data collecting systems. PQRI uses claims information for nearly all of the reported data elements, and over 120 measures are calculated from the submitted data. Of course, not all measures apply to all physicians; for example, a pediatrician will not have a measurable mammography rate. However, nearly every specialty has applicable measures in the PQRI data set. In a manner similar to Meaningful Use, physicians receive a "bonus" payment from CMS just for reporting the data as of 2011, but after 2014, physicians who fail to report will begin paying a penalty based on a percentage of their Medicare payments. Most observers expect the recording requirements to increase with time to include more clinical data elements from the EMR. The goal of the program is to have a standardized reporting approach for measures that can be used to determine physicians' costs and quality performance for the most important clinical conditions.
- **Performance-based incentives for providers**–although not obvious, physicians and other healthcare providers have lived with an incentive-based healthcare system for decades. Incentives developed

during the 1960s with the advent of Medicare and Medicaid were targeted at ensuring access to care, and so the practitioner's volume of services was important for optimizing reimbursement. During the last two decades or so, the focus on incentives has become cost, and lower cost providers are often more successful at maintaining the volume of patients required to ensure profitability. That approach led to lapses in quality of care as measured by several process and outcome statistics (e.g., NCQA's HEDIS measures) and have caused healthcare reform laws to produce a shift in the payment framework to require certain performance levels, as well as cost reductions, to balance the value-based purchasing requirements of the PPACA. Thus, providers must be able to focus on cost and at the same time improve quality on several standard metrics, a feat that can be very difficult without changing practice patterns and becoming more efficient and effective. Additionally, CMS in particular, but many commercial payers as well, are experimenting with bundled payments, in which a single payment is made to a business entity to fund all resources needed to provide care for an episode, including physicians' fees. Thus, integrated healthcare systems that control all resources for providing care will have a distinct competitive advantage.

- **Patient-Centered Medical Home (PCMH)**–long a dream of primary care physicians, the PCMH appears to have become a popular concept for the healthcare delivery system. Sia and Tonniges of the American Academy of Pediatrics (AAP) introduced the term "medical home" in 1967,[1] and by 1977 the Council on Pediatric Practice had adopted the approach as AAP policy.[2] Initially the concept described the primary care physician as a single source of medical information about a patient but the PCMH has evolved to include a partnership approach with families to provide team-based primary health care that is accessible, family-centered, coordinated, comprehensive, continuous, compassionate, and culturally effective. The AAP's 2002 operational definition specifies 37 activities that should occur within a medical home.[3] The Institute of Medicine (IOM) took notice of the medical home in in 1996,[4] and the use of the medical home mantra was adopted by the American Academy of Family Medicine, which in 2002 conducted a study that launched efforts to develop a strategy to transform the specialty of family medicine to meet the needs of patients through coordinated primary care services. The resulting report,

*The Future of Family Medicine: A Collaborative Project of the Family Medicine Community–The Future of Family Medicine Project,*[5] promotes the concept that every American should have a personal medical home that serves as the focal point through which all individuals receive their acute, chronic, and preventive medical care services. In short, primary care physicians are now assuming greater importance in the healthcare delivery system, which may seem incongruous in an era of increasing specialization in medicine, but the new model of the medical home is different from that originally conceived nearly 30 years ago. The complexity of medical care, particularly for patients with complicated chronic conditions, requires teamwork, and so care teams have become the keystone of contemporary primary care. The physician-centered healthcare system is no longer the norm in clinical care, but patients are now assuming the focus of attention. Indeed, physicians are expected to be good team members, not just team leaders. The PCMH is a leading example of this new paradigm, with primary care teams now including nurses, therapists, social workers, and several other health professionals to coordinate care among many sites, often with multiple payment sources, and typically complex care plans.

- **Multiple sources of health information**–PCMH teams are frequently challenged by patients who have conflicting opinions regarding their health care, and these patients have new sources of information, particularly via the Internet. The second most frequent category of search terms on the Web relates to health issues, and this ready source of potentially erroneous data can interfere with an individual's evidence-based care plan. The PCMH must develop a sufficient level of trust with each patient to ensure that patients will always use the PCMH as the ultimate resource, but the ubiquity of information on the Internet makes the search for health information irresistible to most people. Thus, patients who are being treated for a complex disorder might find a Web page that advocates nonmedical treatments that can conflict with the care plan, or worse, some advice that undermines the patient's willingness to complete recommended therapy. In any event, these widely available information resources can prove to be a factor in any care management program.
- **Disparities in care based on diversity**–the United States is a true melting pot with many different ethnicities, some of which might

have misconceptions regarding health care. Often, a lack of cultural sensitivity can create anxiety or misunderstanding regarding health recommendations, with resulting lack of adherence and subsequent treatment failures.[6] Public payers like CMS are directing increased attention to these disparities in care and outcomes to gain insight into the differences and eliminate diversity as a cause of poorer outcomes.

• **Health Information Exchanges (HIEs)**–although not a new phenomenon, HIEs have become increasingly important in the reform era. With greater standardization of protocols for data exchange, interfacing disparate systems has become more straightforward, making large, interactive data repositories more feasible. HIEs represent an evolutionary product of the Community Health Information Networks (CHINs) of the 1980s and 90s, in which communities and regions attempted to create repositories for their areas that allowed sharing of clinical information among multiple providers. Since communication and security protocols were relatively immature at that time, CHINs enjoyed only scattered success, but their current form, Regional Health Information Organizations (RHIOs), are often the nexus for development of HIEs. Thus, some states are connecting preexisting RHIOs to create a distributed database system to satisfy HIE specifications set by the Office of the National Coordinator of Health Information Technology (ONCHIT), the agency set up by Congress to encourage the dissemination of computer technology throughout the healthcare industry. HIEs promise to collect data from multiple sources, such as electronic medical records (EMRs), billing systems, pharmacy benefit management systems, laboratory systems, and others, to create an accessible electronic medical record that providers can use from literally anywhere with an Internet connection. Thus, a primary care physician can immediately see the results of an emergency department visit the night before a follow-up appointment in the office. Having access to nearly all sources of patient information can enable each patient's medical home provider to better manage care and reduce the chance of complications due to conflicting treatments. Although HIEs are in the early stages of deployment, nearly every state in the US has a project to create these useful systems.

• **Ownership of patient clinical record information**–although most physicians have always had a sense of ownership of the records that they create for patients, the true "legal" owner of the record has always been the individual for whom it was created. All of the new methods of recording patient data electronically, though, have created a new dynamic in patient engagement in managing the medical record. Newer commercial systems have been created over the past few years that allow individuals to create personal health records (PHRs). PHRs can be paper-based, but the current iteration that has attracted a great deal of attention is the electronic PHRs such as those listed in **Table 8-1**. PHRs are not the same as electronic health records (EHRs), since they typically allow only the patient to enter and access data, but the fact that PHRs are created in software systems that are interoperable, it is highly likely that the data recorded in the PHR will ultimately be shared with EHRs. PHRs can contain a diverse range of data but usually include information about:

- Family history
- Social history (e.g., smoking, alcohol consumption, etc.)
- Allergies
- Adverse drug reactions
- Diseases, both acute and chronic
- Hospitalizations and surgical procedures
- Laboratory and imaging results
- Immunizations
- Medications–current and prior, including self-administered and over-the-counter medications
- Activities of daily living (ADLs)

**Table 8-1** Examples of personal health record programs

| Resource | Website |
| --- | --- |
| Google Health | http://www.google.com/health |
| Microsoft HealthVault | http://www.healthvault.com |
| WebMD Health Record | http://www.webmd.com/phr |
| Healthy Circles | https://www.healthycircles.com/p_consumer_portal.aspx |
| AHIMA MyPHR | http://www.myphr.com/ |
| MyHealtheVet | http://www.myhealth.va.gov/ |

Some PHRs are developing the ability to check the information in the personal record for drug interactions and to tailor educational materials presented to the patient based on the presence of specific diseases or risk factors. Many systems also now provide interfaces to facilitate secure communication between physicians and patients. One of the key functions of the PHR, however, is the ability of most systems to restrict access to the individual's data based on specific criteria that may be set by the individual user. For example, if a patient did not want a primary care physician to be aware of a psychiatric condition, the patient can restrict related information in the PHR to prevent the physician's access to that specific information. Patients are rapidly becoming not just the legal owners of their records, but the physical owners as well. An important implication of this level of control is the trusting relationship that must be developed between the patient and physician to ensure that the physician can access all of the information necessary to act optimally in the patient's best interest.

# NEW FINANCIAL AND QUALITY REALITIES

The CMS Notice of Proposed Rule Making (NPRM) for Accountable Care Organizations (ACOs) was published in the Congressional Record in March of 2011, and the relationship of quality and cost in the reform era became clearer, at least from the standpoint of CMS. Perhaps one of the most innovative and controversial elements of the PPACA is the Accountable Care Organization, and the level of integration required by this new business entity will likely cause a significant number of organizations to defer formation of an ACO until after the first three-year contract period. However, the melding of quality and cost into the VBP model has begun to permeate the commercial sector as well. The CMS model for attenuating payments through shared savings and quality adjustments will certainly constitute an important new paradigm, and so will be examined in more detail in this section.

Although the PPACA has numerous features that are part of the healthcare reform movement, ACOs have proven to be the most important new model of reimbursement. The law outlines the basics of the model, but the NPRM specifies the parameters for the program that must be operationalized by participating providers, termed "ACO providers," in the NPRM. ACO providers can be any primary care practitioner, such as a family physician, pediatrician, internist, or certain types of advanced practice nurses. An ACO is defined by this group of ACO providers and other suppliers of services (e.g., hospitals, specialty physicians, and others involved in patient care) who work together to coordinate care for the patients they serve in Medicare Parts A and B (the existing fee-for-service [FFS] Medicare program). Care coordination and management will be key approaches to ensuring that the ACO provides seamless, high-quality care, and in many cases, these approaches will require reorganization of existing health practices. Not only will patient care be coordinated through the ACO, but payments to providers will also be the responsibility of the new organization. Patient engagement will be mandatory in this type of arrangement, and the NPRM indicates that patients and caretakers must be involved in decision making, which requires appropriate education and processes for ensuring that patients and caretakers are true partners in care decisions.

"ACO professionals" are defined in the NPRM and PPACA as physicians, advanced practice nurses, and physicians' assistants, and the NPRM indicates that a number of types of organizations with these ACO professionals may participate as ACOs:

- Group practice arrangements
- Networks of individual practices
- Partnerships or joint venture arrangements between hospitals and ACO professionals
- Hospitals employing ACO professionals
- Other Medicare providers and suppliers as determined by the Secretary, including certain critical access hospitals

ACOs must have their own tax identification numbers (TINs), which means that they must be actual business entities within the states in which they operate, and they must apply for approval as an ACO to CMS. To participate in the Shared Savings Program, providers must form or join an ACO and apply to CMS. An existing ACO will **not** be automatically accepted into the Shared Savings Program. If accepted, they would serve at least 5000 Medicare patients for a three year contract term. The Shared Savings Program is designed for Medicare Parts A and B, and at least for the foreseeable future will be designed for a fee-for-service (FFS) environment.

In its application, the ACO must describe its plans to establish a governing body that represents providers, suppliers, and Medicare beneficiaries, as well as a system for monitoring and reporting on the care it delivers according to a monitoring and reporting plan that includes claims analysis and evaluation of specific financial and clinical quality data defined by a list of 65 quality measures that are included in Appendix I. Reports will be required quarterly and annually, and ACOs will be expected to conduct site visits at physicians' offices and survey beneficiaries regarding their care.

## FINANCIAL MODELS

The Medicare Shared Savings Plan, which is the basis for incentives for ACOs and providers, provides ACO providers with potential returns based on their performance on cost containment and clinical improvement initiatives. However, each ACO's beneficiary population would have a benchmark savings target set by CMS that represents the total expected Medicare FFS expenditures for the ACO population if the current trend in cost growth was not modified by the ACO. **Figure 8-1** provides a graphical representation of the use of the benchmark and target savings for the ACO.

The graph in Figure 8-1 illustrates the method by which CMS would calculate savings for the program. CMS actuaries would calculate the rate of increase in costs demonstrated by the population selected for the

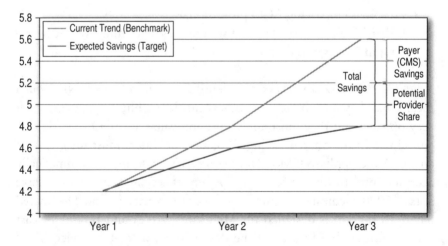

**FIGURE 8-1** Benchmark and target savings concepts for ACOs

ACO, which represents the benchmark for the ACO beneficiary population. CMS then would also determine a target savings rate, which would be used to determine the total savings expected by the quality improvement and cost attenuation activities of the ACO. The benchmark is set during the first year of the contract (benchmark year) and updated each year thereafter to account for changes in the patient population as ACO members enter and leave the ACO population as they change primary care providers. Shared savings are distributed during the second and third years of the contract (performance years), and the ACO shares in a percentage of the savings based on the organization's gainsharing arrangement with CMS. The NPRM outlines two different possible arrangements that are detailed in **Table 8-2**. The NPRM has a complex method of calculating the shared savings that an ACO may receive that takes into account the level of savings, quality performance, and the use of providers from Federally Qualified Health Clinics (FQHCs) and Rural Health Clinics (RHCs) to perform a portion of the primary care clinical services.

The NPRM proposes to implement both a one-sided risk model in which only savings are shared in the first two years and then both savings and losses in the third year, and a two-sided risk model in which the ACO shares in savings and losses for all three years. ACOs may opt for either of the models, but the upside (i.e., the percentage of savings shared) is

**Table 8-2** Tracks for shared savings for ACOs

| Element | One-sided model | Two-sided model |
| --- | --- | --- |
| Maximum sharing rate[a] | 52.5% | 65% |
| Quality scoring[b] | Sharing rate up to 50% based on quality performance | Sharing rate up to 60% based on quality performance |
| FQHC/RHC incentives[c] | Up to 2.5 percentage points | Up to 5 percentage points |
| Minimum savings rate[d] | Variable by population | 2% |
| Minimum loss rate[e] | None | 2% |
| Maximum sharing cap[f] | Payment capped at 7.5% of ACO's benchmark | Payment capped at 10% of ACO's benchmark |

## Table 8-2 Tracks for shared savings for ACOs (*continued*)

| Element | One-sided model | Two-sided model |
|---|---|---|
| Shared savings | Savings shared start once minimum savings rate is exceeded<br><br>Share in savings net of 2% threshold<br><br>Up to 52.5% of net savings up to cap based on quality performance | Savings shared once minimum savings rate is exceeded<br><br>Up to 65% of gross savings up to cap based on quality performance |
| Shared losses | None | Shared losses start once the minimum loss rate is exceeded.<br><br>Cap on the amount of losses to be shared phased in over three years starting at 5% in year 1; 7.5 % in year 2; and 10 % in year 3.<br><br>Losses in excess of the annual cap would not be shared.<br><br>Actual amount of shared losses would be based on final sharing rate that reflects ACO quality performance and any additional incentives for including FQHCs and/or RHCs (1 minus final sharing rate). |

a  Maximum sharing rate is the maximum percentage of the shared savings for which the ACO will be eligible.

b  Quality scoring modifies the actual amount of savings based on a scoring system that equates relative performance on the 65 ACO quality measures.

c  FQHC/RHC incentives add up to 5 percentage points based on the level of participation of Federally Qualified Health Clinics (FQHCs) and Rural Health Clinics (RHCs) in the ACO's patient care.

d  Minimum savings rate is the minimum percentage of savings that must be surpassed before sharing of savings will start. Thus, if the MCO's total savings is $1 million, then the ACO will begin sharing the savings with CMS after the first $20,000 of the savings (which will be retained by CMS).

e  Minimum loss rate applies only to the shared losses for the two-sided model, in which the first 2% of losses are not paid back by the ACO; thus, if the MCO's total losses are $1 million, the ACO will be required to pay $980,000 since the first $20,000 is discounted.

f  Maximum sharing cap is the percentage of the ACO's benchmark that limits the total amount of savings that may be shared with the ACO. For example, if a two-sided ACO's benchmark is $50 million, then the maximum sharing amount that can be shared is $5 million.

higher for the two-sided model. The one-sided model may work better for organizations with less experience managing financial risk, like some physician-driven organizations that have traditionally been paid in a fee-for-service system, while the two-sided model provides a higher return for more experienced provider groups, like capitated Independent Practice Associations (IPAs) that are ready to share both gains and losses. These arrangements are different from traditional capitation arrangements, however, in that the ACO's downside risk is capped at a percentage of its benchmark, although the ACO must find a way of ensuring that any losses are covered, such as through a withhold or reinsurance.

The NPRM establishes a minimum savings rate (MSR), which is a percentage of the benchmark that ACO expenditure savings must exceed in order for an ACO to qualify for shared savings in any given year. The MSR is based on the premise that in any given time period, some improvement in quality and/or cost may be based on random variation alone, and so the ACO should not receive a return for that proportion of the savings. ACOs in the one-sided risk program that have smaller populations and consequently more chance of random variation as a factor in expenditures would have a larger MSR, and those with larger populations and less expected variation in expenditures would have a smaller MSR. The rates are statistically determined based on confidence intervals that vary according to population size as shown in **Table 8-3**. As shown in the table, ACOs in the one-sided risk program that have relatively smaller populations (e.g., 5,000 – 5,999) have a much higher MSR than those with larger populations. ACOs that contract for the two-sided approach will have a flat 2% minimum savings rate. Thus, if an ACO meets quality standards and achieves savings exceeding the MSR, the ACO would share in savings, based on a calculation that modulates the shared savings based on the quality score of the ACO. ACOs may be able to share in savings at a higher rate if a certain number of primary care visits are completed with either a Federally Qualified Health Center or Rural Health Clinic during the performance year.

ACOs that meet quality and cost performance standards will be eligible to share in the savings that is below the benchmark calculated actuarially for the population and also above the MSR. After the MSR is passed,

**Table 8-3** Population sizes and minimum savings rate for one-sided risk model

| Number of beneficiaries | CI | MSR (low end) | MSR (high end) |
| --- | --- | --- | --- |
| 5000 – 5999 | 90% | 3.9% | 3.6% |
| 6000 – 6999 | 90% | 3.6% | 3.4% |
| 7000 – 7999 | 90% | 3.4% | 3.2% |
| 8000 – 8999 | 90% | 3.2% | 3.1% |
| 9000 – 9999 | 90% | 3.1% | 3.0% |
| 10000 – 14999 | 90% | 3.0% | 2.7% |
| 15000 – 19999 | 90% | 2.7% | 2.5% |
| 20000 – 49999 | 95% | 2.5% | 2.2% |
| 50000 – 59999 | 99% | 2.2% | 2.0% |
| > 60000 | | 2.0% (minimum allowed) | |

the ACO begins to share in savings based on the calculated quality performance score. This score has a fairly complex underlying derivation, which will be described shortly. CMS is encouraging ACOs to adopt the two-sided approach, and even those ACOs that choose the one-sided approach will be required to convert to the two-sided approach by the third year of the contract (the second performance year). However, the incentive for adopting the two-sided approach is quite appealing: the maximum sharing percentage (MSP) (i.e., the maximum percentage of the savings that the ACO may receive based on performance criteria) for two-sided ACOs is 60%, while the MSP for one-sided ACOs is only 50%. Two-sided model ACOs would receive shared savings for the first dollar after the minimum savings rate is achieved, while the one-sided model ACOs would share on savings after a 2% threshold is met, although small ACOs in rural or underserved communities are exempt from this threshold.

Just as the MSR adjusts for random variation in improvements, losses in two-sided ACOs are adjusted as well. First, a 2% threshold must be passed for losses to be incurred by the ACO; thus, two-sided model ACOs would assume the losses after the per capita cost per beneficiary exceeds 2% of the benchmark. Fortunately, ACO quality scores will serve to attenuate the losses, with higher quality scores serving to lower the amounts of the losses that the ACO must cover. Additionally, to further encourage participation in the two-sided contracts, the NPRM includes shared loss caps of 5% of the benchmark in the first year of the Shared Savings Program, 7.5% in the second year, and 10% in the third year.

## QUALITY REPORTING AND IMPROVEMENT

Most organizations lack the infrastructure for improving quality measures in the ACO environment proposed in the NPRM. Recognizing that fact, CMS will only require ACOs to report the quality measures in 2012 in order to earn the maximum sharing rate of 60% for two-sided model ACOs and 50% for one-sided model ACOs. In subsequent years, ACOs will be compared with peers, and based on the percentile in which they fall for each of the metrics, they will receive a score that is translated into a percentage used to calculate the final share of the savings, as shown in **Table 8-4**. The NPRM proposes to use percentile rankings of ACO peers to determine point assignments for each quality measure, and so an organization that ranked in the top tenth percentile for a measure would receive 2 points for that metric; in the second decile (80–90 percentile) the ACO would receive 1.85 points, and so on. The points are summed across all measures and then divided by the total number of possible points (2 points per measure multiplied by 65 measures, or 130 possible points) to produce a percentage that is used to calculate the final gain share for the ACO. A sample calculation is shown in **Table 8-5**.

### Table 8-4  Proposed quality point determination after 2012

| Performance level | Points |
| --- | --- |
| 90+ percentile FFS/MA Rate or 90+ percent | 2 |
| 80+ percentile FFS/MA Rate or 80+ percent | 1.85 |
| 70+ percentile FFS/MA Rate or 70+ percent | 1.7 |
| 60+ percentile FFS/MA Rate or 60+ percent | 1.55 |
| 50+ percentile FFS/MA Rate or 50+ percent | 1.4 |
| 40+ percentile FFS/MA Rate or 40+ percent | 1.25 |
| 30+ percentile FFS/MA Rate or 30+ percent | 1.1 |
| < 30 percentile FFS/MA Rate or <30 percent | 0 |

**Table 8-5** Sample quality score calculation

| Measure | Description (Appendix I) | Percent of benchmark (ACO performance) | Points (From Table E-4) | Possible points (2 points per measure for 65 measures) |
|---|---|---|---|---|
| 1 | Clinician/group CAHPS: Getting timely care, appts, and info | 53% | 1.40 | 2 |
| 2 | Clinician/group CAHPS: How well your doctors communicate | 89% | 1.85 | 2 |
| 3 | Clinician/group CAHPS: Helpful, courteous, respectful office staff | 42% | 1.25 | 2 |
| 4 | Clinician/group CAHPS: Patients' rating of doctor | 69% | 1.55 | 2 |
| 5 | Clinician/group CAHPS: Health promotion and education | 92% | 2.00 | 2 |
| ... | ... | ... | ... | ... |
| 65 | Monthly INR for beneficiaries on warfarin | 84% | 1.85 | 2 |
| | Average percentage of monthly intervals in which Part D beneficiaries with claims for warfarin do not receive an INR test during the measurement period | | | |
| TOTALS | | | 103.6 | 130 |
| Percentage | | | 79.6% | |

## Example 8-1 Calculation of ACO gain share for each performance year

The Oncall Care Associate (OCA) Accountable Care Organization finished its first performance year with the scores shown in Figure 8-5. OCA's quality scores generated a quality percentage of 79.6%, and because of effective care management, OCA met the cost targets for its first performance year, and as a two-sided model ACO, the organization qualified for 60% of the savings that it generated during the year. The actual shared percentage, however, is calculated as follows:

*Actual shared savings = Quality Percent × Shared Savings Rate = 0.796 × 0.6 = 0.478*

The shared savings that OCA may expect to receive is thus **47.8%** of the amount that the organization generated in savings.

In 2012, ACOs (both one- and two-sided models) will only be required to report the measures correctly to be able to share in the gains made during the year. ACOs will be eligible for the maximum sharing rate (60% for the two-sided model and 50% for the one-sided model) if they generate sufficient savings and successfully report the required quality measures. This concession allows newly formed ACOs a grace period as they start up their operations and learn to better manage care, collect data, and coordinate transitions between providers.

Importantly, all of the measures that are required in Appendix I are standardized metrics that are used by CMS and other payers and accrediting agencies to assess quality in healthcare organizations through such programs as the physician quality reporting system (PQRS), the electronic health records reporting program, and others. Thus, organizations that have already begun focusing on quality are familiar with these metrics and likely have programs in place to improve performance using these standardized statistics. As noted in the Appendix, these nationally recognized measures fall into five key domains: patient experience, care coordination, patient safety, preventive health, and at-risk population/frail elderly health. Those ACOs that successfully report the quality measures required under the Shared Savings Program would thus be simultaneously eligible for the PQRS bonus.

Some potential ACOs may already have sufficient infrastructure, including capability to receive and distribute FFS payments, repaying shared losses, and having a governance structure that fits that ACO regulations. In those situations, the organization will not be required to form a new entity to apply to be recognized as an ACO. Without those features, however, an organization must either restructure or form a new entity.

# HEALTH INFORMATION TECHNOLOGY (HIT)

The growth in HIT in the past decade has been unprecedented. Increasing numbers of healthcare providers are using electronic health records (EHRs), not just in response to Meaningful Use requirements[7] to qualify for incentives, but also because physicians have been inexorably moving away from independent private practices and into employment arrangements[8] that require use of EHRs. Consumer use of computer technology to find medical information in the "cloud" (Internet) has surged over the past decade as well, and more consumers expect physicians to be conversant with contemporary information sources and to communicate using electronic means.[9] The NPRM requires that ACOs must ensure that 50% of PCPs in the organization qualify for Meaningful Use by the second performance year (year three of the initial contract) to qualify for ACO status (i.e., at least 50% of primary care physicians will use EHRs for patient care within three years for the majority of patient care documentation, order entry, and medication prescribing). Most ACOs will likely have nearly all physicians using EHRs within that timeframe, more to effectively deploy care management and cost reduction than to simply meet the requirements to maintain ACO membership.

This increased volume of electronically accessible patient information will not only make medical records more legible, but the information that now requires costly paper chart audits will be greatly expedited, making quality analysis and reporting less expensive, more accurate, and thus more effective.

On the other hand, the measures that are used to evaluate quality are based heavily on claims data, and in some cases Medicare beneficiaries may not want certain providers to have access to all available information in their claims. The NPRM requires that ACOs allow beneficiaries to opt out of having their claims information shared with physicians and the ACO, but those beneficiaries may still be included in the calculations of the ACO's quality and cost measures. Of course, this lack of information may seriously hamper the ACO's ability to implement quality and cost containment programs, and so the ACO must have a robust way of tracking patients to find patients who are noncompliant, making EHRs even more important for success.

As ACOs begin operating and working to effect changes in patient care, the need for HIT as the backbone of these efforts is unquestioned.

Most organizations that will become the most effective in this new paradigm will quickly implement or expand deployment of an effective clinical information system.

## ROLE OF DMAIC AS A QUALITY IMPROVEMENT STRATEGY

There is little doubt that quality improvement has assumed an important role in health care, and the federal ACO rules represent just one representation of how quality has now become a salient issue in provider compensation. However, those healthcare organizations that are most successful in the new paradigm will recognize the significance of advanced performance improvement approaches to achieve sustainability. First, quality scoring is based not on an ACO's absolute performance, but rather on its quality performance relative to that of its peers. Thus, if the ACO implements quality improvements just like those of its peers, then even improvements in quality scores may not move it sufficiently in relationship to competitors to raise its quality scores. For example, if all ACOs within a cohort improved their performance on "Measure 38: Diabetes Mellitus: Tobacco Non Use–Tobacco use assessment and cessation," then each ACO's position on the distribution relative to others would not change, relative ranking percentiles would not change, and each ACO's quality score would not change. Instead, this method of measurement requires that ACOs that hope to compete successfully must find ways of achieving gains that surpass those of competitors (i.e., gains like those realized through Lean Six Sigma programs). DMAIC becomes one of the key strategic tools in the new world of reform.

Secondly, commercial vendors are modifying their compensation programs to model the PPACA reform act, including bundled payment programs and quality requirements for provider performance. Providers must quickly learn methods of improving patient care, including throughput and access to care, in order to meet the new conditions for practice. The time for slow, incremental change has passed. Consumers and payers alike are demanding more value from the healthcare system, and traditional methods of change lack the focus and power of Lean Six Sigma and the DMAIC approach. Healthcare providers of the 21st century will not be sustainable without effective means of managing patients across the continuum of care, and the risk models that are evolving demand an aggressive approach to ensuring that patients receive evidence-based, rapidly available medical services in appropriate settings.

Finally, DMAIC provides the basis for rapid cycle interventions, as well as more sustained quality programs. An organization that bases its quality program on the Lean Six Sigma approach has the concentration and, with appropriate leadership, the motivation to achieve high performance goals that may take much longer in other organizations that lack the resolve and dedication required for LSS. The case studies in Chapter 7 demonstrated the power of LSS in practice, and the ability of healthcare organizations to excel using this approach has been shown repeatedly. Now the only question remains–when will you start?

# DISCUSSION QUESTIONS

1. The United States Congress passed the Patient Protection and Affordable Care Act in 2010. What provision in the Act has become the most important in melding quality and cost?
2. Define value-based purchasing. How does this concept translate into practice through the PPACA?
3. Meaningful Use was designed to improve physician use of EHRs and EMRs. Why is this initiative important to value-based purchasing?
4. Describe the concept of ICD-10 coding. Why is it important to improving information analysis in health care?
5. Performance based payment systems are relatively new in health care. Describe how these programs influence quality in health care.
6. Describe the Patient Centered Medical Home. Why is it important for improving care and implementing reform?
7. What sources do people have for healthcare information? How do these multiple sources present challenges to healthcare providers?
8. How does population diversity complicate the job of healthcare providers? How will this challenge affect the ability of providers to meet the requirements of healthcare reform?
9. What are health information exchanges? How will they change the delivery of health care?
10. Who owns patient clinical information? How will control of access to patient information change in the future?

11. What is an Accountable Care Organization? What major role do these organizations play in the reform era?

12. Describe the Shared Savings Program. How will these new incentives change healthcare delivery?

13. Describe the quality measures required for ACOs. How are they organized in domains? How will performance on these measures be scored?

14. How do quality scores affect reimbursement in an ACO?

15. Health information technology is expected to be a linchpin for healthcare reform. Why is HIT important?

16. How does LSS create the environment necessary for success in the reform era?

## REFERENCES

1. Sia, C., Tonniges, T.F., Osterhus, E., & Taba, S. (2004). History of the medical home concept. *Pediatrics.* 113(5 Suppl),1473–1478.

2. American Academy of Pediatrics, Council on Pediatric Practice. (1977). Fragmentation of health care services for children. News and Comment. *Pediatrics*, Supplement, April.

3. Medical Home Initiatives for Children with Special Needs Project Advisory Committee. (2002). The medical home. *Pediatrics*, 110, 184–186.

4. Institute of Medicine (US), & Donaldson, M. (1996). *Primary care: America's health in a new era.* Washington, DC: National Academy Press.

5. Kahn, N. (2004). The future of family medicine: A collaborative project of the family medicine community, Future of Family Medicine Project Leadership Committee, *Annals of Family Medicine*, 2, S3-S32. Retrieved from http://www.annfammed.org/cgi/content/abstract/2/suppl_1/s3.

6. Shavers, V.L., & Brown, M.L. (2002). Racial and ethnic disparities in the receipt of cancer treatment. *Journal of the National Cancer Institute*, 94(5), 334–57, Retrieved from http://jnci.oxfordjournals.org/content/94/5/334.full.

7. Office of the National Coordinator for Health Information Technology. (2011). *Meaningful use and EHRs.* Retrieved from http://healthit.hhs.gov/portal/server.pt?open=512&objID=2996&mode=2.

8. Beaulieu, D. (2010). MGMA: Hospital-employment trend rippling out to affect compensation. *Fiercepracticemanagement.com.* Retrieved from http://www.fiercepracticemanagement.com/story/mgma-65-percent-established-physicians-hired-hospital-owned-practices-2009/2010-06-04.

9. Coalition for Healthcare Communication. (2011). Do not track: Coming soon–A mobile device near you? Retreived from http://www.cohealthcom.org/2011/03/04/pew-survey-confirms-importance-of-internet-to-consumers/.

# Quality Measures for Accountable Care Organizations

| # | Domain | Title/Description | Measure Steward | Method | Type |
|---|--------|------------------|-----------------|--------|------|
| 1 | Pt/caregiver experience | Clinician/Group CAHPS: Getting timely care, appointments, and info | NQF #5 | Survey | Experience of care |
| 2 | Pt/caregiver experience | Clinician/Group CAHPS: How well your doctors communicate | NQF #5 | Survey | Experience of care |
| 3 | Pt/caregiver experience | Clinician/Group CAHPS: Helpful, courteous, respectful office staff | NQF #5 | Survey | Experience of care |
| 4 | Pt/caregiver experience | Clinician/Group CAHPS: Patients' rating of doctor | NQF #5 | Survey | Experience of care |
| 5 | Pt/caregiver experience | Clinician/Group CAHPS: Health promotion and education | NQF #5 | Survey | Experience of care |
| 6 | Pt/caregiver experience | Clinician/Group CAHPS: Shared decision making | NQF #5 | Survey | Experience of care |
| 7 | Pt/caregiver experience | Medicare Advantage CAHPS: Health status/functional status | NQF #6 | Survey | Experience of care |
| 8 | Care coordination/ transitions | Risk-standardized, all condition readmission: The rate of readmissions within 30 days of discharge from an acute care hospital for assigned ACO beneficiary population | CMS | Claims | Outcome |
| 9 | Care coordination/ transitions | 30 day post discharge physician visit | CMS | GPRO reporting tool | Process |

| | | | | GPRO reporting tool | |
|---|---|---|---|---|---|
| 10 | Care coordination/ transitions | Medication reconciliation: Reconciliation after discharge from an inpatient facility Percentage of patients aged 65 years and older discharged from any inpatient facility (e.g., hospital, skilled nursing facility, or rehabilitation facility) and seen within 60 days following discharge in the office by the physician providing ongoing care who had a reconciliation of the discharge medications with the current medication list in the medical record documented | NQF #554 | | Process |
| 11 | Care coordination/ transitions | Care transition measure: Unidimensional self-reported survey that measures the quality of preparation for care transitions; Namely: 1. Understanding one's self-care role in the posthospital setting 2. Medication management 3. Having one's preferences incorporated into the care plan | NQF #228 | Survey | Experience of care |
| 12 | Care coordination | Ambulatory sensitive conditions Admissions: Diabetes, short-term complications (AHRQ Prevention Quality Indicator [PQI] #1) All discharges of age 18 years and older with ICD-9-CM principal diagnosis code for short-term complications (ketoacidosis, hyperosmolarity, coma), per 100,000 population | NQF #272 | Claims | Outcome |
| 13 | Care coordination | Ambulatory sensitive conditions Admissions: Uncontrolled diabetes (AHRQ Prevention Quality Indicator [PQI] #14) All discharges of age 18 years and older with ICD-9-CM principal diagnosis code for uncontrolled diabetes, without mention of a short-term or long-term complication, per 100,000 population | NQF #638 | Claims | Outcome |

*(continued)*

| # | Domain | Title/Description | Measure Steward | Method | Type |
|---|--------|-------------------|-----------------|--------|------|
| 14 | Care coordination | Ambulatory sensitive conditions Admissions: Chronic obstructive pulmonary disease (COPD) (AHRQ Prevention Quality Indicator [PQI] #5) All discharges of age 18 years and older with ICD-9-CM principal diagnosis code for COPD, per 100,000 population | NQF #275 | Claims | Outcome |
| 15 | Care coordination | Ambulatory sensitive conditions Admissions: Congestive heart failure (AHRQ Prevention Quality Indicator [PQI] #8) All discharges of age 18 years and older with ICD-9-CM principal diagnosis code for CHF, per 100,000 population | NQF #277 | Claims | Outcome |
| 16 | Care coordination | Ambulatory sensitive conditions Admissions: Dehydration (AHRQ Prevention Quality Indicator [PQI]#10) All discharges of age 18 years and older with ICD-9-CM principal diagnosis code for hypovolemia, per 100,000 population | NQF #280 | Claims | Outcome |
| 17 | Care coordination | Ambulatory sensitive conditions Admissions: Bacterial pneumonia (AHRQ Prevention Quality Indicator [PQI] #11) All nonmaternal discharges of age 18 years and older with ICD-9-CM principal diagnosis code for bacterial pneumonia, per 100,000 population | NQF #279 | Claims | Outcome |

| | | | | | |
|---|---|---|---|---|---|
| 18 | Care coordination | Ambulatory sensitive conditions Admissions: Urinary infections (AHRQ Prevention Quality Indicator [PQI]#12) All discharges of age 18 years and older with ICD-9-CM principal diagnosis code of urinary tract infection, per 100,000 population | NQF #281 | Claims | Outcome |
| 19 | Care coordination/ Information systems | % all physicians meeting Stage 1 HITECH meaningful use requirements | CMS | GPRO data collection tool / EHR Incentive Program reporting | Process |
| 20 | Care coordination/ Information systems | Ambulatory sensitive conditions Admissions: Bacterial pneumonia (AHRQ Prevention Quality Indicator [PQI] #11) All nonmaternal discharges of age 18 years and older with ICD-9-CM principal diagnosis code for bacterial pneumonia, per 100,000 population | CMS | GPRO data collection tool / EHR Incentive Program reporting | Process |
| 21 | Care coordination/ Information systems | Percent of PCPs using clinical decision support | CMS EHR Incentive Program core measure | GPRO data collection tool / EHR Incentive Program reporting | Process |

*(continued)*

| # | Domain | Title/Description | Measure Steward | Method | Type |
|---|--------|------------------|-----------------|--------|------|
| 22 | Care coordination/ Information systems | Percent of PCPs who are successful electronic prescribers under the eRx Incentive Program | CMS EHR Incentive Program core measure | GPRO data collection tool / eRx Incentive Program reporting | Process |
| 23 | Care coordination/ Information systems | Patient registry use | CMS EHR Incentive Program menu set measure | GPRO data collection tool | Process |
| 24 | Care coordination/ Information systems | Healthcare acquired conditions composite: <br>• Foreign object retained after surgery <br>• Air embolism <br>• Blood incompatibility <br>• Pressure ulcer, Stages III and IV <br>• Falls and trauma <br>• Catheter-associated UTI <br>• Manifestations of poor glycemic control <br>• Central line associated blood stream infection (CLABSI) <br>• Surgical site infection | CMS (HACs), NQF #531 (AHRQ PSI) | Claims or CDC National Healthcare Safety Network | Outcome |

| | | | | | |
|---|---|---|---|---|---|
| | | • AHRQ Patient Safety Indicator (PSI) 90 Complication/Patient safety for selected indicators (composite)<br>  • Accidental puncture or laceration<br>  • Iatrogenic pneumothorax<br>  • Postoperative DVT or PE<br>  • Postoperative wound dehiscence<br>  • Decubitus ulcer<br>  • Selected infections due to medical care (PSI 07: Central venous catheter-related bloodstream infection)<br>  • Postoperative hip fracture<br>  • Postoperative sepsis | | | |
| 25 | Patient safety | Healthcare-acquired conditions: CLABSI bundle | NQF #298 | Claims or CDC National Healthcare Safety Network | Process |
| 26 | Preventive health | Influenza immunization:<br>Percentage of patients aged 50 years and older who received an influenza immunization during the flu season (September through February) | PQRS Measure #110 EHR Incentive Program—Clinical quality measure NQF #41 | GPRO data collection tool | Process |

(continued)

| # | Domain | Title/Description | Measure Steward | Method | Type |
|---|--------|-------------------|-----------------|--------|------|
| 27 | Preventive health | Pneumococcal vaccination: Percentage of patients aged 65 years and older who have ever received a pneumococcal vaccine | PQRS Measure #111 EHR Incentive Program—Clinical quality measure NQF #44 | GPRO data collection tool | Process |
| 28 | Preventive health | Mammography screening: Percentage of women aged 40 through 69 years who had a mammogram to screen for breast cancer within 24 months | PQRS Measure #112 EHR Incentive Program—Clinical quality measure NQF #31 | GPRO data collection tool | Process |
| 29 | Preventive health | Colorectal cancer screening: Percentage of patients aged 50 through 75 years who received the appropriate colorectal cancer screening | PQRS Measure #113 EHR Incentive Program—Clinical quality measure NQF #34 | GPRO data collection tool | Process |

| # | Category | Description | Program/Measure | Tool | Type |
|---|---|---|---|---|---|
| 30 | Preventive health | Cholesterol management for patients with cardiovascular conditions:<br>The percentage of members 18–75 years of age who were discharged alive for AMI, coronary artery bypass graft (CABG) or percutaneous coronary interventions (PCI) of the year prior to the measurement year, or who had a diagnosis of ischemic vascular disease (IVD) during the measurement year and the year prior to the measurement year, who had each of the following during the measurement year; LDL-C screening LDL-C control (< 100 mg/dL) | EHR Incentive Program–Clinical quality measure NQF #75 | GPRO data collection tool | Process & outcome |
| 31 | Preventive health | Adult weight screening and follow up:<br>Percentage of patients aged 18 years and older with a calculated BMI in the past six months or during the current visit documented in the medical record AND if the most recent BMI is outside parameters, a follow-up plan is documented<br>Parameters:<br>Age 65 and older BMI ≥ 30 or < 22;<br>Age 18-64 BMI ≥ 25 or < 18.5 | PQRS Measure #128 EHR Incentive Program–Clinical quality measure NQF #421 | GPRO data collection tool | Process |
| 32 | Preventive health | Blood pressure measurement:<br>Percentage of patient visits with blood pressure measurement recorded among all patient visits for patients aged > 18 years with diagnosed hypertension | PQRS Measure #TBD EHR Incentive Program–Clinical quality measure NQF 13 | GPRO data collection tool | Process |

(continued)

| # | Domain | Title/Description | Measure Steward | Method | Type |
|---|--------|-------------------|-----------------|--------|------|
| 33 | Preventive health | Tobacco use assessment and tobacco cessation Intervention: Percentage of patients who were queried about tobacco use; Percentage of patients identified as tobacco users who received cessation intervention | PQRS Measure #TBD EHR Incentive Program– Clinical quality measure NQF 28 | GPRO data collection tool | Process |
| 34 | Preventive health | Depression screening: Percentage of patients aged 18 years and older screened for clinical depression using a standardized tool and follow up plan documented | PQRS Measure #134 NQF 418 | GPRO data collection tool | Process |
| 35 | At risk population– diabetes | Diabetes composite (all or nothing scoring): Hemoglobin A1c control (< 8%) Low density lipoprotein (< 100) Blood pressure < 140/90 Tobacco nonuse Aspirin use | NQF #575, 64, 61, 28, TBD | GPRO data collection tool | Process & outcome |
| 36 | At risk population– diabetes | Diabetes mellitus: Hemoglobin A1c control (< 8%) Percentage of patients aged 18 through 75 years with diabetes mellitus who had most recent hemoglobin A1c less than 8.0% | EHR Incentive Program– Clinical quality measure NQF #575 | GPRO data collection tool | Outcome |

| # | Population | Measure | PQRS/NQF | Data collection | Type |
|---|---|---|---|---|---|
| 37 | At risk population – diabetes | Diabetes mellitus: Low density lipoprotein (LDL-C) Control in diabetes mellitus. Percentage of patients aged 18 through 75 years with diabetes mellitus who had most recent LDL-C level in control (less than 100 mg/dl) | PQRS Measure #2 EHR Incentive Program–Clinical quality measure NQF #64 | GPRO data collection tool | Outcome |
| 38 | At risk population – diabetes | Diabetes mellitus: Tobacco nonuse. Tobacco use assessment and cessation | PQRS Measure #TBD EHR Incentive Program–Clinical quality measure NQF #28 | GPRO data collection tool | Process |
| 39 | At risk population – diabetes | Diabetes mellitus: Aspirin use. Daily aspirin use for patients with diabetes & cardiovascular disease | NQF TBD | GPRO data collection tool | Process |
| 40 | At risk population – diabetes | Diabetes mellitus: Hemoglobin A1c poor control (> 9%): Percentage of patients aged 18 through 75 years with diabetes mellitus who had most recent hemoglobin A1c greater than 9.0% | PQRS Measure #1 EHR Incentive Program–Clinical quality measure NQF #59 | GPRO data collection tool | Outcome |

(continued)

| # | Domain | Title/Description | Measure Steward | Method | Type |
|---|--------|-------------------|-----------------|--------|------|
| 41 | At risk population – diabetes | Diabetes mellitus: High blood pressure control in diabetes mellitus: Percentage of patients aged 18 through 75 years with diabetes mellitus who had most recent blood pressure in control (less than 140/90 mmHg) | PQRS Measure #3 EHR Incentive Program–Clinical quality measure NQF #61 | GPRO data collection tool | Outcome |
| 42 | At risk population – diabetes | Diabetes mellitus: Urine screening for microalbumin or medical attention for nephropathy in diabetic patients Percentage of patients aged 18 through 75 years with diabetes mellitus who received urine protein screening or medical attention for nephropathy during at least one office visit within 12 months | PQRS Measure #119 EHR Incentive Program–Clinical quality measure NQF #62 | GPRO data collection tool | Process |
| 43 | At risk population – diabetes | Diabetes mellitus: Dilated eye exam in diabetic patients Percentage of patients aged 18 through 75 years with a diagnosis of diabetes mellitus who had a dilated eye exam | PQRS Measure #117 EHR Incentive Program–Clinical quality measure NQF #55 | GPRO data collection tool | Process |

| 44 | At risk population–diabetes | Diabetes mellitus: Foot exam The percentage of patients aged 18 through 75 years with diabetes who had a foot examination | PQRS Measure #163 EHR Incentive Program–Clinical quality measure NQF #56 | GPRO data collection tool | Process |
|----|----|----|----|----|----|
| 45 | At risk population–heart failure | Heart failure: Left ventricular function (LVF) assessment Percentage of patients aged 18 years and older with a diagnosis of heart failure who have quantitative or qualitative results of LVF assessment recorded | PQRS Measure #198 NQF #79 | GPRO data collection tool | Process |
| 46 | At risk population–heart failure | Heart failure: Left ventricular function (LVF) testing Percentage of patients with LVF testing during the current year for patients hospitalized with a principal diagnosis of heart failure (HF) during the measurement period | PQRS Measure #228 CMS | GPRO data collection tool | Process |
| 47 | At risk population–heart failure | Heart failure: Weight measurement Percentage of patient visits for patients aged 18 years and older with a diagnosis of heart failure with weight measurement recorded | PQRS Measure #227 NQF #82 | GPRO data collection tool | Process |
| 48 | At risk population–heart failure | Heart failure: Patient education Percentage of patients aged 18 years and older with a diagnosis of heart failure who were provided with patient education on disease management and health behavior changes during one or more visit(s) within 12 months | PQRS Measure #199 NQF #82 | GPRO data collection tool | Process |

*(continued)*

| # | Domain | Title/Description | Measure Steward | Method | Type |
|---|--------|-------------------|-----------------|--------|------|
| 49 | At risk population–heart failure | Heart failure: Beta-blocker therapy for left ventricular systolic dysfunction (LVSD)<br>Percentage of patients aged 18 years and older with a diagnosis of heart failure who also have LVSD (LVEF < 40%) and who were prescribed beta-blocker therapy | PQRS Measure #8<br>EHR Incentive Program–Clinical quality measure NQF #83 | GPRO data collection tool | Process |
| 50 | At risk population–heart failure | Heart failure: Angiotensin-converting enzyme (ACE) inhibitor or angiotensin receptor blocker (ARB) Therapy for left ventricular systolic dysfunction (LVSD)<br>Percentage of patients aged 18 years and older with a diagnosis of heart failure and LVSD (LVEF < 40%) who were prescribed ACE inhibitor or ARB therapy | PQRS Measure #5<br>EHR Incentive Program–Clinical quality measure NQF #81 | GPRO data collection tool | Process |
| 51 | At risk population–heart failure | Heart failure: Warfarin therapy for patients with atrial fibrillation<br>Percentage of all patients aged 18 and older with a diagnosis of heart failure and paroxysmal or chronic atrial fibrillation who were prescribed warfarin therapy | PQRS Measure #200<br>EHR Incentive Program–Clinical quality measure NQF #84 | GPRO data collection tool | Process |

| # | Domain | Measure | Reference | Data collection tool | Type |
|---|---|---|---|---|---|
| 52 | At risk population–coronary artery disease | Coronary artery disease (CAD) composite: All or nothing scoring<br>Oral antiplatelet therapy prescribed for patients with CAD<br>Drug therapy for lowering LDL cholesterol<br>Beta-blocker therapy for CAD patients with prior myocardial infarction (MI)<br>LDL Level < 100 mg/dl<br>Angiotensin-converting enzyme (ACE) inhibitor or angiotensin receptor blocker (ARB) therapy for patients with CAD and diabetes and/or left ventricular systolic dysfunction (LVSD) | NQF #67, 74, 70, 64, 66 | GPRO data collection tool | Process & outcome |
| 53 | At risk population–coronary artery disease | Coronary artery disease (CAD):<br>Oral antiplatelet therapy prescribed for patients with CAD<br>Percentage of patients aged 18 years and older with a diagnosis of CAD who were prescribed oral antiplatelet therapy | PQRS Measure #6 EHR Incentive Program–Clinical quality measure NQF #67 | GPRO data collection tool | Process |
| 54 | At risk population–coronary artery disease | Coronary artery disease (CAD): Drug therapy for lowering LDL cholesterol<br>Percentage of patients aged 18 years and older with a diagnosis of CAD who were prescribed a lipid-lowering therapy (based on current ACC/AHA guidelines)<br>The LDL-C treatment goal is < 100 mg/dl; Persons with established coronary heart disease (CHD) who have a baseline LDLC 130 mg/dl should be started on a cholesterol-lowering drug simultaneously with therapeutic lifestyle changes and control of nonlipid risk factors (National Cholesterol Education Program [NCEP]) | PQRS Measure #197 EHR Incentive Program–Clinical quality measure NQF #74 | GPRO data collection tool | Process |

*(continued)*

| # | Domain | Title/Description | Measure Steward | Method | Type |
|---|---|---|---|---|---|
| 55 | At risk population–coronary artery disease | Coronary artery disease (CAD): Beta-blocker therapy for CAD patients with prior myocardial infarction (MI) Percentage of patients aged 18 years and older with a diagnosis of CAD and prior MI who were prescribed beta-blocker therapy | PQRS Measure #7 EHR Incentive Program–Clinical quality measure NQF #70 | GPRO data collection tool | Process |
| 56 | At risk population–coronary artery disease | Coronary artery disease (CAD): LDL level < 100 mg/dl | CMS | GPRO data collection tool | Outcome |
| 57 | At risk population–coronary artery disease | Coronary artery disease (CAD): Angiotensin-converting enzyme (ACE) inhibitor or angiotensin receptor blocker (ARB) therapy for patients with CAD and diabetes and/or left ventricular systolic dysfunction (LVSD) Percentage of patients aged 18 years and older with a diagnosis of CAD who also have diabetes mellitus and/or LVSD (LVEF < 40%) who were prescribed ACE inhibitor or ARB therapy | PQRS Measure #118 NQF #66 | GPRO data collection tool | Process |
| 58 | At risk population–hypertension | Hypertension (HTN): Blood pressure Control Percentage of patients with last BP < 140/90 mmHg | PQRS Measure #TBD EHR Incentive Program–Clinical quality measure NQF #18 | GPRO data collection tool | Outcome |

| # | Population | Measure | ID | Data Source | Type |
|---|---|---|---|---|---|
| 59 | At risk population–hypertension | Hypertension (HTN): Plan of care — Percentage of patient visits for patients aged 18 years and older with a diagnosis of HTN with either systolic blood pressure ≥ 140 mmHg or diastolic blood pressure ≥ 90 mmHg with documented plan of care for hypertension | PQRS Measure #TBD NQF #17 | GPRO data collection tool | Process |
| 60 | At risk population–COPD | Chronic obstructive pulmonary disease (COPD): Spirometry evaluation — Percentage of patients aged 18 years and older with a diagnosis of COPD who had spirometry evaluation results documented | PQRS Measure #51 NQF #91 | GPRO data collection tool | Process |
| 61 | At risk population–COPD | Chronic obstructive pulmonary disease (COPD): Smoking cessation counseling received | CMS | GPRO data collection tool | Process |
| 62 | At risk population–COPD | Chronic obstructive pulmonary disease (COPD): Bronchodilator therapy based on FEV1 — Percentage of patients aged 18 years and older with a diagnosis of COPD and who have an FEV1/FVC less than 70% and have symptoms who were prescribed an inhaled bronchodilator | PQRS Measure #52 NQF #102 | GPRO data collection tool | Process |
| 63 | At risk population–frail elderly | Falls: Screening for fall risk — Percentage of patients aged 65 years and older who were screened for fall risk at least once within 12 months | NQF #101 | GPRO data collection tool | Process |
| 64 | At risk population–frail elderly | Osteoporosis management in women who had a fracture — Percentage of women 65 years and older who suffered a fracture and who had either a bone mineral density (BMD) test or prescription for a drug to treat or prevent osteoporosis in the 6 months after the date of fracture | NQF #53 | Claims | Process |
| 65 | At risk population–frail elderly | Monthly INR for beneficiaries on warfarin — Average percentage of monthly intervals in which Part D beneficiaries with claims for warfarin do not receive an INR test during the measurement period | NQF #555 | Claims | Process |

# DMAIC Terms
# and Definitions

**Acceptance region**   The region of values for which the null hypothesis is accepted.

**Accuracy**
1. The degree to which an indicated value matches the actual value of a measured variable.
2. In process instrumentation, degree of conformity of an indicated value to a recognized accepted standard value, or ideal value.

**Affinity chart/diagram**   A tool for organizing large quantities of information from many people. It is often used with brainstorming and other creative thinking activities to consolidate ideas into coherent subgroups. The ideas are usually written on sticky notes, then categorized into groupings of similar ideas.

**Agile management**   The ability to thrive under conditions of constant and unpredictable change by seeking to achieve rapid response to customer needs. Agile management also emphasizes the ability to quickly reconfigure operations–and strategic alliances–to respond rapidly to unforeseen shifts in the marketplace, which in the healthcare industry of the 21st century, is critical to survival. Healthcare leaders now recognize the need for applying other principles, like "mass customization," to satisfy unique customer requirements but maintaining the efficiencies of a mass production operation.

**Alpha risk**   The probability of accepting the alternate hypothesis when, in reality, the null hypothesis is true.

**Alternate hypothesis**   A tentative explanation that indicates that an event does not follow a chance distribution; a contrast to the null hypothesis.

**"As-Is" process map**   A process map that depicts a process as it is, currently. "As-is" process maps are usually characterized by several input options, bottlenecks and multiple handoffs, inspections, and rework loops. This diagram is the starting point to understanding how a process is currently functioning and where opportunities for improvement might be found.

**Assignable (special) cause**   A source of variation that is nonrandom; a change in the source ("VITAL FEW" variables) will produce a significant change of some magnitude in the response (dependent variable), e.g., a correlation exists; an assignable cause is often signaled by an excessive number of data points outside a control limit and/or a nonrandom pattern within the control limits; an unnatural source of variation; most often economical to eliminate.

**Assignable variation**   Variations in data that can be attributed to specific causes.

**Attribute**   A characteristic that may take on only one value (e.g., 0 or 1).

**Attribute data**   Numerical information at the nominal level; subdivision is not conceptually meaningful; data that represents the frequency of occurrence within some discrete category (e.g., 24 defective X-ray images).

**Autonomation (Jidoka)**  "Automation with a human touch"; design of a process so that machines automatically inspect items as they are produced, with the ability to notify humans if a defect is detected and stop production of the item or service. In the Toyota Production System, this concept is extended to include all workers on the production line or involved in the process. Each worker is empowered to stop production if a defect is discovered, which has particular applicability in the healthcare delivery system to prevent harm to patients.

**Background variables**  Variables that are of no experimental interest and are not held constant. Their effects are often assumed insignificant or negligible, or they are randomized to ensure that contamination of the primary response does not occur.

**Baka yoke**  Literally to design a process to be foolproof; a process or a machine is designed so that the only way it can be performed or used is the correct way. This type of process design generally involves a warning if the process or machine produces a nonstandard condition. Healthcare applications have been concentrated on failure Mode and effects analyses, using such tools as Pareto analysis.

**Baseline measures**  Data that reflect the performance level that exists at the beginning of an improvement project, before any solutions are initiated.

**Best practice**  A completed project or other evidence that is particularly valuable for use in other situations. As evidence for a particular practice increases, it can reach the level of a best (or leading) practice when it demonstrates consistently superior outcomes and low variation.

**Beta risk**  The probability of accepting the null hypothesis when, in reality, the alternate hypothesis is true.

**Black Belt**  The leader of the team responsible for applying the Six Sigma process.

**Calibration** Determination of the experimental relationship between the quantity being measured and the output of the device that measures it; where the quantity measured is obtained through a recognized standard of measurement.

**Cause and effect diagram (Ishikawa)** Brainstorming tool used for proposing root-causes (the "bones of the fish") for a specific effect (the "head of the fish"). Typically used in combination with the affinity diagram to determine the major categories and with the "5 Whys" technique in order to help people understand the root cause.

**Cellular manufacturing** A process design approach in which equipment and workstations are arranged to facilitate small-lot, continuous-flow production. In a manufacturing context, a "cell" is designed so that all operations necessary to produce a component or subassembly are performed in close proximity, thus allowing for quick feedback between operators when quality problems and other issues arise. Cross training workers in a manufacturing cell ensures that each worker in the cell can assume responsibility for any step.

**Center line** The line on a statistical process control chart that represents the characteristic's central tendency.

**Central tendency** Numerical average (e.g., mean, median, and mode); center line on a statistical process control chart.

**Chaku-chaku** "Load-load" in Japanese. A method of implementing single-piece flow in which the operator proceeds from machine to machine, taking a part from the previous operation and loading it in the next machine, then taking the part just removed from that machine and loading it in the following machine.

**Champion** Person responsible for the logistical and business aspects of a Six Sigma project. Champions select and scope projects that are aligned with the corporate strategy, choose and mentor the right people for the project, and remove barriers to ensure the highest levels of success.

**Charter** Team document defining the context, specifics, and plans of an improvement project; includes business case, problem and goal statements, constraints and assumptions, roles, preliminary plan, and scope. The charter is to be reviewed with the project sponsor to ensure alignment and revised or refined periodically throughout the DMAIC process based on data.

**Checksheet** Forms, tables, or worksheets developed as part of the project plan for use in data collection to standardize data collection.

**Common cause (random) variation** Random variation inherent in a process due to process design, variability in human or machine performance, or other uncontrolled variation. This form of variation is usually harder to eliminate than special cause variation and will require changes to the process.

**Confidence level** The probability that a random variable x lies within a defined interval.

**Confidence limits** The two values that define the confidence interval.

**Confounding** Allowing two or more variables to vary together so that it is impossible to separate their unique effects.

**Consumers' risk** Probability of accepting a product or service when, in fact, it should have been rejected (same as beta risk).

**Continuous data** Any quantity measured on a continuous scale that can be infinitely divided; primary types include time, dollars, size, weight, temperature, and speed; also referred to as "variable data."

**Continuous-flow production** Implementation of "just in time" techniques to reduce setup times, slash work-in-progress inventory, reduce waste, minimize nonvalue-added activities, improve throughput, and reduce cycle time. Continuous-flow production typically involves use of "pull" signals to initiate production activity, in contrast to work-order ("push") systems in which production scheduling typically is based on forecasted demand rather than actual demand. In many "pull" systems, a customer order or delivery date triggers completion of the process, which in turn cascades messages backwards in the process to force replenishment of components required for upstream inventory to prepare for subsequent production.

**Continuous random variable**   A random variable that can assume any value continuously in some specified interval.

**Control**
1. The state of stability, normal variation and predictability.
2. The process of regulating and guiding operations and processes using quantitative data.

**Control chart**   A graphical rendition of a characteristic's performance across time in relation to its natural limits and central tendency.

**Control specifications**   Specifications called for by the product being manufactured or service being delivered.

**Controlled variable**
1. The variable that the control system attempts to keep at the set point value. The set point may be constant or variable.
2. The part of a process to be controlled (flow, level, temperature, pressure, etc.).
3. A process variable that is to be controlled at some desired value by means of manipulating another process variable.

**Correlation**   A measure of the degree to which two variables (such as thunder and lightning or tardiness and/or low productivity) are related (i.e., the extent to which they move together). Used to quantify the strength of the relationship between the two variables, correlation does not necessarily imply a cause and effect relationship. For example, daily high temperatures and ice cream sales would tend to be correlated, and so it is reasonable to conclude that hotter weather causes people to buy more ice cream. However, the conclusion cannot be made that hot weather always causes people to buy more ice cream, since other variables may affect that outcome.

**Cost of poor quality (COPQ)**   Financial metrics that measure the impact of quality problems (internal and external failures) in the process; sources of costs include labor and material costs for handoffs, rework, waste or scrap, inspection, and other nonvalue-added activities.

**Cpk**   A statistic that indicates how well a design tolerance compares with the normal process variation (defined as +/-3s) that also accounts for the difference between the process target and the actual process mean. Cpk values vary between zero and 2, with higher values being desirable. Cpk values of 1.33 are considered a minimum acceptable process capability, indicating a sigma level of 3; higher Cpk values approach Six Sigma capability of 3.4 defective units per million opportunities.

**Criteria matrix**   Decision support tool used when potential choices must be weighted against key factors (e.g., cost, ease to implement, impact on customer). Encourages use of facts, data, and clear business objectives in the decision-making process.

**Critical-to-quality (CTQ, Critical Y)**   The element of a process or practice that has a direct impact on its perceived quality from the customer's perspective; features that customers consider the most important in a product or service.

**Cross-functional teams**   Multidisciplinary and interdepartmental teams of employees who represent a cross section of disciplines and/or different process segments who participate on ad hoc teams to deal with a specific problem or perform a specific task.

**Customer**   Any internal or external person or organization that receives the output (product or service) of a process.

**Customer requirements**  The needs and expectations of the customer, translated into measurable terms and used in process improvement to ensure compliance with customers' needs. Customer requirements define CTQ (critical-to-quality) attributes that become the Y values in the six sigma equation.

**Cycle time**  In industrial engineering, the time between completion of two discrete units of production. For example, in health care the cycle time of a surgical unit would be the number of cases performed per hour or some other time unit. The goal of a process is for cycle time to equal takt time, which indicates single piece flow.

**Dashboard**  A set of metrics, usually not more than five or six, that provide an "at-a-glance" summary of a Six Sigma project's status. Every participant in a Six Sigma deployment – from the CEO to a factory floor worker – should have his or her own dashboard with function- and level-appropriate data summaries.

**Data**  Factual information used as a basis for reasoning, discussion, or calculation; often refers to quantitative information.

**Data collection plan**  A structured approach to identifying the required data to be collected and the approach to collecting it; typically performed during the Measure Phase of a DMAIC project. The data collection plan includes: the measure, the measure type, data type, operational definition, and the sampling plan if new data is necessary.

**Defect**  Source of customer dissatisfaction. Eliminating defects provides cost and quality benefits.

**Defects Per Million Opportunities (DPMO)**  Calculation used in Six Sigma initiatives to show how much "better" or "worse" a process is by indicating the number of defects in a process per one million opportunities to have a defect. The measure is calculated by the following equation:

$$DPMO = \frac{Number\ of\ defects}{Number\ of\ opportunities} \times 1,000,000$$

An issue for consideration is how many opportunities should be in the denominator. For example, if foreign bodies left in situ post operatively is the measure of interest, then the number of procedures in which at least one foreign body was left in the surgical site would be in the denominator and the total number of surgical procedures would be in the denominator. On the other hand, the number of DPMO in a run of 1,000 medical invoices would be calculated as follows: each invoice has 20 fields that are completed, and 1,000 bills are in each batch. Thus, the number of opportunities is $20 \times 1,000$ or 20,000. If 50 bills have three errors each, then the number of defects is 150 and the DPMO is calculated as follows:

$$\text{DPMO} = (150/20{,}000) \times 1{,}000{,}000 \text{ or}$$
$$\text{DPMO} = 7{,}500$$

The best guideline for counting opportunities is to use only those that directly affect the use of the final output. Thus, in the billing example, any of the errors would result in rejection of the claim. However, if half of those errors would not result in a rejected claim, then the calculations becomes:

$$\text{DPMO} = (75/20{,}000) \times 1{,}000{,}000 \text{ or}$$
$$\text{DPMO} = 3{,}750$$

**Degrees of freedom (df)**   The number of independent measurements available for estimating a population parameter

**Density function**   The function that yields the probability that a particular random variable takes on any one of its possible values.

**Dependent variable**   A Response Variable (e.g., y is the dependent or "Response" variable where Y=f [X]).

**Deployment flowchart**   A map or graphical view of the steps in a process shows the sequence as it moves across departments, functions, or individuals. This type of process map shows "hand-offs" and the groups involved. It is also known as a functional or cross-functional flowchart or map.

**Descriptive statistics**   A statistical profile of the collected data that includes measures of averages, variance, and standard deviation, that help define the level of performance and variation in the sample or population.

**Design for Six Sigma (DFSS)**   Application of six sigma tools to product or service development with the goal of "designing in" six sigma performance capability.

**Deviation**   The difference between the value of a specific variable and some desired value, usually a process set point.

**Discrete random variable**   A random variable that can assume values only from a definite number of discrete values.

**Distributions**   Tendency of large numbers of observations to group themselves around some central value with a certain amount of variation or "scatter" on either side.

**DMADV (Design, Measure, Analyze, Design, Verify)**   The framework for applying Six Sigma tools for designing new products, services, and processes. DMADV is used when:

- A service is not yet in existence. An existing product, service, or process has been optimized, but still does not meet the level of customer specifications or a Six Sigma level.

**DMAIC (Define, Measure, Analyze, Improve, and Control)**   Framework for continued improvement that is systematic, scientific, and fact based. This closed-loop process eliminates unproductive steps, often focuses on new measurements, and applies technology for improvement.

**Efficiency**   Measure related to the quantity of resources used in producing the output of a process (e.g., cost of the process, total cycle time, resources consumed, cost of defects, scrap, and/or waste); links primarily to company profitability.

**Effectiveness**   Measures related to how well the process output(s) meets the needs of the customer (e.g., on-time delivery, adherence to specifications, service experience, accuracy, value-added features, customer satisfaction level); links primarily to customer satisfaction.

**Experiment**   A test under defined conditions to determine an unknown effect; to illustrate or verify a known law; to test or establish a hypothesis.

**Experimental error**   Variation in observations made under identical test conditions. Also called residual error. The amount of variation that cannot be attributed to the variables included in the experiment.

**External failure**   A failure characterized by customers receiving defective units that have passed completely through the process.

**Factors**   Independent variables.

**Five Whys**   A root cause analysis technique that consists of asking "Why" five times in order to delve deeply into each potential cause. "Why" is asked until the root cause is revealed.

**First-pass yield**   The percent of finished product or service units that meet all quality-related specifications at a critical test point in the process. This metric assesses the yield that results from the first time through the process, prior to any rework, and it is calculated as the percent of output that meets target-grade specifications after the first time through the process.

**Five (5) Ss**
   **Sort**   To clearly distinguish the needed from the unneeded
   **Straighten**   Keeping needed items in the correct place to allow for easy and immediate retrieval
   **Shine**   Keeping the workplace swept and clean
   **Standardize**   Consistently applying 6S methods in a uniform and disciplined manner
   **Sustain**   Making a habit of maintaining established procedures
   **OR** 5S   Refers to the five Japanese words:
   **seiri**   Eliminating everything not required for the work being performed
   **seiton**   Efficient placement and arrangement of equipment and material
   **seison**   Tidiness and cleanliness

**seiketsu** Ongoing, standardized, continually improving seiri, seiton, seison

**shitsuke** Discipline with leadership

**Fixed effects model** Experimental treatments are specifically selected by the researcher. Conclusions only apply to the factor levels considered in the analysis. Inferences are restricted to the experimental levels.

**Flexible manufacturing systems** Automated manufacturing equipment and/or cross-trained work teams that can accommodate small-lot production of a variety of product or part configurations. In a service environment, FMS connotes cross training for improved productivity and use of small teams in "microsystems."

**Flow** The progressive achievement of tasks along the value stream so that a product or service proceeds through each step of the process with no stoppages, waste, or backflows.

**FMEA (Failure modes and effects analysis)** A procedure used to identify and assess risks associated with potential product or process failure modes.

**Force field analysis** A list of the factors that support an issue juxtaposed with a list of factors that oppose the issue. Support factors are listed as "Driving Forces" and opposing factors are listed as "Restraining Forces."

**Frequency distribution** The pattern or shape formed by the group of measurements in a distribution.

**Gauge** A device or process by which measurements are taken (also spelled "Gage").

**Gauge R&R (Gauge repeatability and reproducibility)** A statistical tool that measures the amount of variation in the measurement system from the device used, the people taking the measurement, the interaction between the device and the person and the error seen from the parts.

**Gantt chart**    A project planning and management tool that displays all the tasks or activities associated with a project or initiative as well as the relationships/dependencies between these tasks. Resources, completion status, timing, and constraints are all shown in the chart.

**Goal statement**    Description of the intended target or desired results of process improvement or design/redesign activities; usually outlined during the Define Phase of a DMAIC project and supported with actual numbers and details once data has been obtained.

**Green Belt**    An individual who supports the implementation and application of Six Sigma tools by way of participation on project teams.

**Handoff**    Any time in a process when one person (or job title) or group passes the item moving through the process to another person; a handoff has the potential to add defects, time, and cost to a process.

**Hawthorne effect**    An increase in worker productivity that results from the psychological stimulus of being temporarily singled out and made to feel important. A group working on a project may be receiving a lot of attention and their performance may temporarily improve; when this attention decreases, the worker motivation may decline resulting in lower productivity.

**Heijunka**    A Japanese word that means "make flat and level," referring to production smoothing, which is a technique used to adapt production to naturally fluctuating customer demand. Customer demand must be met within preferred delivery times, but customer demand is uneven, necessitating interventions on the part of managers to smooth demand as much as possible.

**Histogram**    Vertical display of a population distribution in terms of frequencies; a formal method of plotting a frequency distribution.

**Homogeneity of variance**    The variances of the groups being contrasted are equal (as defined by statistical test of significant difference).

**Hoshin kanri (Policy deployment)**   Alignment of strategy with improvement initiatives to achieve strategic objectives. Visual matrix diagrams are used to select three to five key objectives and translate them into specific projects deployed at the front-line customer level. Targets for these objectives are established and used to measure progress toward goals.

**Human factors**   Human capabilities and limitations to the design and organization of the work environment; primarily attributed to errors, but also a consideration in the design of workflow and processes. The study of human factors can help identify operations susceptible to human error and improve working conditions to reduce fatigue and inattention.

**Hypothesis statement**
1. In Six Sigma or project management, a complete description of the suspected causes of a process problem.
2. In statistics, a testable statement of a relationship between factors, such as a cause and effect relationship.

**Impact/effort matrix**   A matrix comparison of different projects plotted along two axes (Y = Impact, X = Effort). The project that demonstrates the highest impact with the lowest effort is determined the best selection.

**Implementation plan**   A project management tool used in the Improve Phase of DMAIC, compiling tools such as stakeholder analysis, FMEA, Poka-yoke, standard operating procedures, and pilot results (if conducted) in a consolidated format.

**Improvement**   In the lean process management system, improvement is a philosophy of maintaining and improving high quality standards that guides activities such as kaizen events. Through innovation and other lean tools, improvement guides workers in the philosophy of the organization to achieve high standards of quality.

**Independent variable**   A controlled variable; a variable whose value is independent of the value of another variable.

**Interaction**  The tendency of two or more variables to produce an effect in combination that neither variable would produce if acting alone.

**Internal rate of return (IRR)**  The annualized effective compounded return rate that can be earned on invested capital (i.e., the yield on the investment). The internal rate of return for an investment is the discount rate that makes the net present value of the investment's income stream total to zero. This metric is used for comparing potential projects. Project planning should strive for a high IRR.

**Interval**  Numeric categories with equal units of measure but no absolute zero point (i.e., quality scale or index).

**Just-in-time (JIT)**  A system for producing and delivering the right items at the right time in the right amounts at the right place in the process.

**Kaikaku**  Radical improvement of an activity to eliminate muda (e.g., by implementing single piece flow in a small space that reduces travel). Also called breakthrough kaizen, flow kaizen, and system kaizen.

**Kaizen**  The systematic, organized improvement of processes by front line staff, using straightforward methods of analysis and improvement. Kaizen can be an immediate approach to continuous, incremental improvement of an activity to create more value with less muda by establishing priorities and empowering employees to use continuous improvement tools to gain immediate results.

**OR**

The philosophy of continuous improvement, that requires every process to be continually evaluated and improved by everyone working on the process. In the TPS, kaizen applies to all aspects of life, not just work.

**Kaizen event**  A defined effort in which a multidisciplinary team plans and implements a significant process change to quickly achieve a quantum improvement in performance.

**Kanban**   A communication tool developed by Taiichi Ohno at Toyota in the "just-in-time" production and control system that authorizes production or movement. Kanban can be a card or signboard or any other authorizing device such as a light or electronic signal that is attached to specific parts in the production line signifying the delivery of a given quantity. The ideal quantity authorized for each kanban is one unit, but in many applications several units might be authorized. For example, a radiology department might authorize several patients simultaneously if several exam rooms are free. The number of circulating or available kanban for a specific unit is determined by the demand rate for the item and the time required to produce or acquire more. Unless demand changes or other circumstances intervene, the number of available kanban generally remains constant to maintain control of the process. However, more efficient single piece flow systems require few, if any, kanban; so the fewer kanban used, the more efficient the process. Kanban operates according to the following rules:

- All movements of production units (e.g., parts, materials, information, patients) occur only as required by a downstream operation. Thus, all manufacturing, production, and procurement activities are ultimately driven by the requirements of the customer.
- Kanban have various formats and content as appropriate for their usage; for example, a kanban for a vendor is different than a kanban for an internal machining operation.

**Kanban signal**   A method of signaling suppliers or upstream production operations when it is time to replenish limited stocks of components or subassemblies in a just-in-time system. In the TPS, kanban signals were cards placed in specific locations to signal the need for more process units at the next step in the process. Contemporary systems often use electronic signals in place of cards or other physical elements.

**Kano analysis**   A graph of how customer satisfaction is affected by a particular problem, change, or other variable. The graph is divided into three regions of customer reactions to the variable: "Dissatisfiers," "Satisfiers," and "Delighters."

**Karoshi**   Death from overwork. A common problem for QI professionals in health care.

**KPIs**  Key performance indicators, or the few vital measurements that show how a business is performing throughout the production process.

**Lead time**  The total time a customer must wait to receive a product or service after placing an order. For example, the wait time in a physician's office would be considered lead time in a lean system environment. When a production system is running at or below capacity, lead time and throughput time are the same. When customer demand exceeds system capability, waiting time is added to the throughput so that lead time exceeds throughput.

**Lean manufacturing or lean production**  The philosophy of the Toyota Production System to continually reducing waste in all areas and in all forms.

**Level scheduling**  The use of scheduling to sequence production units in a repetitive pattern to smooth variations in the rate of customer demand.

**Life cycle costing**  The identification, evaluation, tracking, and analysis of actual costs for each service or product from the point of initial research and development through the final product or service and after-service support.

**Line balancing**  Achievement of smooth production flow and 100% capacity utilization by equalization of cycle times for relatively small process units using proper allocation of human and physical resources.

**Line charts**  Charts used to track performance without relationship to process capability or control limits.

**Lower control limit**  A horizontal line plotted on a control chart that represents the lower process limit capabilities.

**Machine availability rate**  The percent of time that equipment is available for use, divided by the maximum time it would be available if there were no downtime for repair or unplanned maintenance. This concept may be applied to other physical resources, such as operating room availability rate, emergency department room availability rate, etc.

**Manufacturing cells**   A configuration of equipment and workstations in a sequence (often U-shaped) to support single-piece flow and flexible deployment of human effort. Manufacturing cells are often designed using tools such as the workflow diagram that positions equipment and other resources in a way that optimizes human interaction and decreases travel and wait time.

**Manufacturing cycle time**   The length of time from the start of production operations for a particular service or product to the completion of all production or service processes for a specific customer or customer order. This time does not include order-entry time or time spent on customization of nonstandard items.

**Master Black Belt**   A teacher and mentor of Black Belts. Provides support, reviews projects, and undertakes larger scale projects.

**Measure**   A numerical representation of observable data. For example, serum sodium level, number of bills sent, rooms cleaned per shift.

**Mixed-model production**   The capability to produce a variety of services or variations of a product that may differ in use of human and physical resources in the same production environment; common situation for healthcare systems (e.g., pathology department that must process a variety of specimens for different customers using similar equipment and the same staff).

**Muda (waste)**   Waste that is targeted for elimination in the lean process management system, including:

1. **Overproduction**–excess production and early production leading to inventories
2. **Waiting**–time spent in anticipation of the next process step
3. **Transportation**–time spent in movement and transportation of production units

4. **Processing**–poor process design
5. **Inventory**–waste associated with inventory (e.g., storage, nonproducing assets)
6. **Motion**–actions of people or equipment that do not add value to the product
7. **Rework**–production of an item or service that must be discarded or requires rework

**Multiple regression**   Quantitative method relating multiple factors to the output of a process. The statistical study of the relationship of a combination of multiple variables (X1 X2 X3...Xn) to a single output Y using least squares estimation for each coefficient of variation.

**Multivoting**   A method of reducing a long list of options to a shorter list by having team members cast votes on the options in multiple voting cycles one after another, dropping the options with the fewest votes at the end of each cycle, until the list is reduced to a manageable size.

**Mura**   Variation.

**Muri**   Excessive burden due to waste or poor design.

**Nagara**   Smooth production flow, ideally single piece flow, with synchronization (balancing) of production processes and maximum utilization of available time, including overlapping of operations where practical. Utilization of level scheduling and line balancing to achieve smooth flow.

**Nemawashi**   The Japanese conduct business meetings differently from other cultures. Nemawashi, which translates to "prior consultation," is a method by which everyone involved in the meeting reviews material and makes conclusions regarding the information. By gaining agreement as much as possible in advance, meetings can conclude with a decision and maintain harmony among attendees. The prior preparation allows people with differing opinions to negotiate their differences before the meeting and reduce wasted time in the meeting.

**Nominal** Unordered categories that indicate membership or nonmembership with no implication of quantity (i.e., number of patients with Caesarean section, number of patients treated for hypertension, etc.)

**Nonconforming unit** A unit that does not conform to one or more specifications, standards, and/or requirements.

**Nonconformity** A condition within a unit that does not conform to some specific specification, standard, and/or requirement; often referred to as a defect; any given nonconforming unit can have the potential for more than one nonconformity.

**Nonvalue-added work** Essential process steps or activities that must be performed in the present system, but do not add value to the product or service. These steps or activities are the target of lean process improvement activities.

**Normal distribution** A continuous, symmetrical density function characterized by a bell-shaped curve (e.g., distribution of sampling averages).

**Null hypothesis** A tentative explanation that indicates that a chance distribution is operating; a contrast to the null hypothesis.

**One-sided alternative** The value of a parameter that has an upper bound or a lower bound, but not both.

**Operational definition** A clear, precise definition of the factor being measured or the term being used; ensures a clear understanding of terminology and the ability to collect data or operate a process consistently.

**Ordinal** Ordered categories (ranking) with no information about distance between each category (i.e., rank ordering of several measurements of an output parameter).

**Output/outcome measures** Measures related to and describing the output of the process or outcome for the customer (e.g., mortality rate, injury rate from medical errors, functional status after surgery).

**Parameter**   A constant defining of a particular property of the density function of a variable.

**Pareto diagram**   A chart that ranks, or places in order, common occurrences. A Pareto chart is a data display tool based on the Pareto Principle; or 80/20 rule. It is used to help bring focus to the specific causes or issues that will have the greatest impact if solved.

**P chart**   Control chart used to plot percent defectives in a sample.

**PDSA cycle (Plan-Do-Study-Act)**   Shewhart's improvement cycle in which a process or system is studied and improvements planned, the improvements are initiated (Do), the results of the intervention are reviewed (Study), and the intervention is then either incorporated into the process or subject to the improvement cycle for another round.

**Poka yoke**   A Japanese term for "mistake proofing" that represents the process of empowering workers at every step in the process to seek defects and stop the defects from proceeding further in the process or allow defects to reach the customer. This concept may also involve creative thinking to develop ways to keep errors from occurring. For example, design of connecting hose ends to prevent an oxygen tube from being plugged into a vacuum outlet or labeling drugs with similar sounding names with exaggerated characters to avoid confusing the two medications.

**Population**   A group of similar items from which a sample is drawn. Often referred to as the universe.

**Power of an experiment**   The probability of rejecting the null hypothesis when it is false and accepting the alternate hypothesis when it is true.

**Precision**   The degree of reproducibility among several independent measurements of the same true value.

**Predictive maintenance**   Practices that seek to prevent unscheduled equipment downtime by collecting and analyzing information on equipment conditions. This analysis is used to predict time-to-failure, conduct planned maintenance, and maintain equipment in good operating condition. In the manufacturing sector, predictive maintenance systems typically measure parameters on machine operations, such as vibration, heat, pressure, noise, and lubricant condition, while in health care, bioengineers monitor machine usage time and test for accuracy in parameters like fluid delivery in IV pumps.

**Primary control variables** The major independent variables used in the experiment.

**Probability** The chance of something happening; the percent or number of occurrences over a large number of trials.

**Probability of an event** The number of successful events divided by the total number of trials.

**Process** A series of steps or actions that lead to a result or output. A set of common tasks that creates a product or service.

**Process average** The central tendency of a given process characteristic across a given amount of time or at a specific point in time.

**Process capability** Statistical measures that summarize how much variation there is in a process relative to customer specifications.

**Process management** The cycle of continuous review, reexamination, and renewal of fundamental work processes that contribute to an organization's performance and productivity.

**Process map** Illustrated description of the steps in a process that concisely diagrams the process flow; enables participants to visualize an entire process and identify areas of strength and weakness.

**Process redesign** Method of restructuring a process that addresses common cause variation using techniques to eliminate nonvalue added or detrimental steps that reduce process performance but do not cause the process to operate outside control limits.

**Process spread**   The range of values that a given process characteristic displays; this particular term most often applies to the range but may also encompass the variance. The spread may be based on a set of data collected at a specific point in time or may reflect the variability across a given amount of time.

**Processing time**   The time a patient is actually engaged in receiving a service or a product is being produced on a production line. Typically, processing time is a small fraction of throughput time and lead time.

**Producers' risk**   Probability of rejecting a lot when, in fact, the lot should have been accepted (same as ALPHA RISK).

**Project**   The focus of performance improvement efforts. A defined work effort characterized by a starting point and an ending point.

**Pull**   A system of cascading production and delivery instructions from downstream to upstream activities in which nothing is produced by the upstream supplier until the downstream customer signals a need. For example, flexible staffing of an emergency department that allows for staff to be sent to the ED when volume is higher.

**Pull system**   A system for controlling workflow priorities in which processes requiring resources receive the resources as needed, using techniques such as kanban and just-in-time production. Contrasted with "push" systems in which material is processed, then pushed to the next stage whether or not it is really needed in the downstream environment.

**QFD (quality function deployment)**   A customer-focused approach to quality improvement in which customer needs (desired product or service characteristics) are analyzed at the design stage and translated into specific product, service, and design requirements for the supplier organization. Targeted customer needs may include product features, cost, durability, appearance, or other product characteristics. QFD involves carefully listening to the customer's needs and translating them into product or service design elements to create the desired customer output.

The quality functions defined by the customer are then deployed throughout the organization by tying incentives and compliance activities directly to the fulfillment of these customer requirements.

**Quick changeover methods** A variety of techniques that reduce equipment setup time and permit faster cycle time (e.g., as in operating room turnaround time).

**R chart** Range control chart; a plot of the difference between the highest and lowest in a sample.

**Random** A sampling technique designed so that each item in the population has an equal chance of being selected; lack of predictability; without pattern.

**Random cause** A source of variation that is random; for example, a change in the source ("trivial many" variables) will not produce a highly predictable change in the response (dependent variable) because a correlation does not exist; random causes cannot be economically eliminated from a process, because the source of variation is inherent in the process; common cause.

**Random sample** One or more samples randomly selected from the universe (population).

**Random variable** A variable that can assume any value from a set of possible values.

**Random variation** Variation in data that results from causes that cannot be pinpointed or controlled.

**Range** The difference between the highest and lowest values in a set of values or "subgroup."

**Ranks** Values assigned to items in a sample to determine their relative occurrence in a population.

**Reject region**   The region of values for which the alternate hypothesis is accepted.

**Representative sample**   A sample that accurately reflects a specific condition or set of conditions within the universe.

**Return on investment (ROI)**   A measure of the financial returns from an investment opportunity, expressed as a percentage. All else being equal, projects with a larger ROI are more attractive investment opportunities.

**Rework loop**   Any instance in a process when the item or data moving through the process must be corrected by returning it to a previous step in the process adding time, cost, and potential for errors and more defects.

**Robust**   Impervious to perturbing influence.

**Rolled throughput yield (RTY)**   The cumulative calculation of defects through multiple steps in a process; calculated as the product of the individual yield at each step (expressed as a percentage). For example, in an 8 step process with each step at 99%, the rolled throughput yield is $.99 \times .99 \times .99 \times .99 \times .99 \times .99 \times .99 \times .99 = 95\%$.

**Root cause analysis (RCA)**   A study of underlying reason(s) for nonconformance within a process; correction of the root cause eliminates the nonconformity.

**Run chart**   A plot of a variable over time with a center line (usually the median of the data set) that demonstrates the trend and provides information about trends, patterns, and special cause variation.

**Sample**   One or more observations drawn from a larger collection of observations or universe (population).

**Sampling bias**   Collecting an unrepresentative "slice" of data that will lead to inaccurate conclusions. For instance, measuring the first five patients seen in the clinic to determine waiting times rather than taking a random sample of patients over a period of time.

**Scatter diagrams**   Charts that plot two variables on a Cartesian graph that allow visual study of the relationship between two variables.

**Scope**   Defines the boundaries of the process; clarifies specifically where the start and end points for improvement reside; defines where and what to measure and analyze; sets the sphere of control of the team working on the project; in general, the broader the scope, the more complex and time-consuming the improvement efforts will be.

**Seiban**   A Japanese management practice taken from the Japanese words "sei," which means manufacturing, and "ban," which means number. A Seiban number is assigned to all parts, materials, and purchase orders associated with a particular customer job, or with a project, that enables a process owner to track everything related with a particular product, service, or customer. Seiban also facilitates setting aside inventory for specific projects or priorities to accommodate nonstandard production or service requests.

**Self-directed natural work teams (SDN)**   Autonomous teams of empowered employees that share a common workspace and/or responsibility for a particular process or process segment. SDN work teams have authority for day-to-day production activities and many supervisory responsibilities, such as job assignments, production scheduling, maintenance, materials purchasing, training, quality assurance, performance appraisals, and customer service.

**Sensei**   A teacher or instructor.

**Setup time**   Work required to change over resources from one item or operation to the next item or operation, often seen as two types:

1. **Internal**–setup work that can be done only when the resource is not actively engaged in performing a service or in a production activity
2. **External**–setup work that can be done concurrently with the resource being used in a service process or in a production activity

## Seven quality tools

- Flowcharts
- Cause-and-effect diagrams
- Check sheets
- Histograms
- Scatter diagrams
- Pareto charts
- Control charts

**"Should Be" process map or flowchart** A depiction of a new and improved version of a process, used in DMAIC projects, where all nonvalue added steps have been removed and based on:

- Everything being done right the first time
- Customer requirements built into the process
- Flexibility to meet multiple customer types or requirements
- Design with "process" vs. "functional" mindset
- Limited handoffs and inspections
- Ease to document, manage, train, and control
- Several possible inputs
- Bottleneck eliminated
- Handoffs, inspection, and rework loops no longer needed

**Sigma value** Metric that indicates how well that process is performing. The higher the sigma value, the better. Sigma measures the capability of the process to perform defect-free work. A defect is anything that results in customer dissatisfaction. Sigma is a statistical unit of measure that reflects process capability. The sigma scale of measure is perfectly correlated to such characteristics as defects-per-unit, parts-per million defective, and the probability of a failure/error.

**Signal** An event or phenomenon that conveys data from one point to another.

**Simple linear regression** The statistical study of the relationship between a single variable X to a single output, fitting a line though a set of data to reduce the variation between actual and predicted performance.

**Single piece flow**   A process design in which service units or products proceed, one complete item at a time, through various operations in design, order taking, and production, without interruptions, backflows, or scrap.

**SIPOC**   SIPOC is a high-level process map that includes Suppliers, Inputs, Process, Outputs, and Customers that define the start and end points of a process. It is used to ensure that the team members are all viewing the process in the same way and inform leadership on the process being improved.

**Six Sigma**   A sigma level indicating a performance level of 3.4 defects per million opportunities (DPMO).

**Spaghetti chart**   A map of the path taken by a specific product or a customer receiving a service as the item or customer travels down the value stream in a lean production organization; so-called because the route typically looks like a plate of spaghetti.

**Special cause**   Same as ASSIGNABLE CAUSE.

**Stable process**   A process that is free of assignable causes (e.g., in statistical control).

**Stakeholder analysis**   Identifies all stakeholders impacted by a project and their anticipated and required levels of support for the project. Typical stakeholders include managers, people who work in the process under study, other departments, customers, suppliers, and finance. Used to identify potential barriers to process improvement efforts.

**Standard deviation**   A statistical index of variability that describes the spread or variation in a data set.

**Standard operating procedure**   A document that compiles all procedures, job tasks, scripts of interactions with customers or others, data collection instructions and forms, and an updated list of resources to be consulted for clarification of procedures. SOPs allow the organization to maintain reproducibility of all aspects of a process improvement across shifts, time periods, and leadership changes.

**Standard work**   A precise description of each work activity specifying cycle time, takt time, the work sequence of specific tasks, and the minimum resources needed to conduct the activity. Standard work details the motion of the worker and the process sequence in producing an item or service. Standard work defines the most muda-free production method, through the best arrangement of resources, the least amount of work in process, with indications of where measurements should be performed for quality and safety. It provides a routine for consistency of an operation and a basis for improvement. A clinical practice guideline is an example of standard work.

**Statistical control**   Process condition that is free of assignable/special causes of variation (e.g., variation in the central tendency and variance, most readily indicated on a control chart).

**Statistical process control (SPC)**   The analysis of measure trends using graphical and statistical methods for measuring, analyzing, and controlling the variation of a process for the purpose of ensuring process performance and continuously improving the process.

**Storyboard**   A visual display outlining the highlights of a project and its components, as well as results. Storyboards are often used to track project progress or for use in presentations to managers and other stakeholders.

**Stratification**   Dividing data sets into groups based on key characteristics to detect patterns that relate to the characteristic. For example, a data set may be stratified into age groups by year or age group to determine the characteristics of each of the groups relative to a variable under study.

**Subgroup**   A logical grouping of objects or events that are used in some SPC charts to sample from a larger population of measurements; samples are randomly selected to decrease bias from assignable or special causes.

**Subprocess**   A section or subset of steps of a larger process. For example, a phlebotomy procedure may be a subprocess of a workup for a child with a fever.

**Systematic sampling**   Sampling method in which elements are selected from the population at a uniform level (e.g., every half-hour, every twentieth item). For example, sampling a process at fixed time intervals represents systematic sampling and ensures each sample will be representative of the process because each time period is represented.

**Takt time**   The available production time divided by the rate of customer demand. Takt time sets the pace of production to match the rate of customer demand. Used to determine targets for improvement of system output.

**Test of significance**   A procedure to determine whether a quantity subjected to random variation differs from a postulated value by an amount greater than that due to random variation alone.

**Throughput time**   Processing and waiting time for performing a service or producing a product.

**Tollgate (or gate)**   A review session that determines whether activities up to that point in a project have been satisfactorily completed. Tollgates are commonly conducted to review critical decisions during a project.

**Total cost of poor quality**   The aggregate cost of service or product failures (e.g., scrap, rework, and warranty costs) as well as expenses incurred to prevent or resolve quality problems (including the cost of inspection).

**Total Productive Maintenance (TPM)**   A comprehensive program to maximize equipment availability in which equipment operators are trained to regularly perform routine maintenance tasks, while technicians and engineers handle more specialized maintenance tasks. The scope of TPM programs includes maintenance prevention (through design or selection of easy-to-service equipment), equipment improvements, preventive maintenance, and predictive maintenance (determining when to replace components before they fail).

**Total Quality Management (TQM)** A multifaceted, company-wide approach to improving all aspects of quality and customer satisfaction—including fast response and service, as well as product quality. TQM begins with top management and ensures that all employees and managers share responsibility and accountability for managing quality.

**Total Quality Control (TQC)** Organized kaizen activities involving everyone in the company—managers and workers—in a totally integrated effort toward improving performance at every level. This improved performance is directed toward satisfying such cross-functional goals as quality, cost, scheduling, manpower development, and new product development. It is assumed that these activities ultimately lead to increased customer satisfaction.

**Tree diagram** A "branching" diagram that is used to break any broad goal into increasingly detailed levels of actions. Often used along with brainstorming or during project management/planning.

**Type I error** Same as ALPHA RISK.

**Type II error** Same as BETA RISK.

**Upper control limit** A horizontal line on a control chart that represents the upper limits of process capability.

**Value** The highest quality for the lowest price. Products or services that meet customers' needs for affordability, availability, and utility.

**Value added activities** Steps or tasks in a process that meet all three criteria defining value as perceived by the external customer:

- Transforms the item/service toward completion
- Customer willing to pay for it
- Done right the first time

**Value stream** The specific activities required to design, order, and provide a specific product or service from concept to final product or service.

**Value stream mapping** Identification of all the specific activities occurring along a value stream for a product or service.

**Variable** A characteristic that may take on different values.

**Variables data** Numerical measurements made at the interval or ratio level; continuous number data.

**Variance**
1. A change in a process or business practice that may alter its expected outcome.
2. A statistical term that is the square of the standard deviation.

**Variation** Any quantifiable difference between individual measurements; such differences can be classified as being due to common causes (random) or special causes (assignable).

**Visual control** The placement in plain view of all tools, parts, production activities, and indicators of production system performance so everyone involved can understand the status of the system at a glance. The use of signals, charts, measurements, diagrams, lights, and signs to clearly define the normal process flow.

**Visual workplace** A visual workplace is a work area that uses visual controls to indicate the structure and function of all processes, to the point that other instruction sets are unneeded. Characteristics of a visual workplace include:

- Physical impediments to effective processing are removed
- Processes are tightly linked and logically ordered
- Tools and fixtures have homes–no searching for lost items
- Information and process elements travel together throughout the process flow Standards are clear and self-explanatory

**Voice of the Business (VOB)**   The stated mission, goals, and business objectives of an organization; specific, documented statements of intent that are the guidelines by which linkages are established between Six Sigma projects and targeted levels of improvement. The Voice of the Business should describe what the business does and how the business intends to accomplish its mission. Combined with the Voice of the Customer, the Voice of the Business plays an important role in defining potential Six Sigma projects.

**Voice of the Customer (VOC)**   A systematic approach for eliciting and analyzing customers' requirements, expectations, level of satisfaction, and areas of concern. The VOC is a key data source in the project selection process.

**X-bar and R chart**   A control chart that uses the values of individual x-values and the range to establish the centerline, upper control limit, and lower control limit.

**Waste**   Needless activities that do not add value to a product or service.

**Work-in-process inventory (WIP)**   The amount or value of all materials, components, and resources representing partially completed products or services; anything on the production sequence that has not been completed.

**Yamazumi**   Meaning literally "to pile in heaps," a yamazumi board is a tool to achieve line balance, with strips of paper or card representing particular tasks. For example, a list of patients in the ED kept on a white board for all to see is one type of yamazumi board.

**Yellow Belt**   A Yellow Belt is any employee who has received introductory training in the fundamentals of Six Sigma. The Yellow Belt gathers data, participates in problem-solving exercises and adds their personal experiences to the exploration process.

**Yield**   Total number of units handled correctly through the process step(s), typically expressed as a percentage. Yield indicates how many items were delivered at the end of the process with no defect.

**Yield improvement**   Percentage reduction in scrap or rejects. For example, if yield of a process, like X-ray film wastage improves from 95% to 98%, then the number of rejects has been reduced by 60% (from 5% waste to 2% waste), which is a yield improvement of 60%.

**Z-score**   Sometimes called "standard scores"; a special application of the transformation rules in which a value within a distribution is divided by the standard deviation of the distribution to provide the proportion of the standard deviation represented by the value. The Z score for a data point indicates how far, and in what direction, that item deviates from its distribution's mean, expressed in units of its distribution's standard deviation.

# Index

## A

AAP (American Academy of Pediatrics),
246–247

abbreviations
avoiding misinterpreting in medication
orders, 11
training program format, 191

acceptance region
defined, 283
in null hypothesis, 129

accountability circle, healthcare, 8–9

Accountable Care Organizations (ACOs)
financial models, 252–257
growth of health information
technology, 260
quality reporting and improvement,
257–259
reimbursement model, 250–252
role of DMAIC, 261–262

Accountable Care Organizations (ACOs),
quality measures for
care coordination, 267–269
care coordination information systems,
269–270
care coordination transitions, 266–267
patient safety, 270
patient/caregiver experience, 266
preventive health, 270–274
at risk population, COPD, 281
at risk population, coronary artery disease,
278–279
at risk population, diabetes, 274–277
at risk population, frail elderly, 281

at risk population, heart failure, 277–278
at risk population, hypertension,
279–280

accuracy
calculating process sigma, 106
cost reduction/revenue enhancement
from, 223
defined, 283
gauge R&R determining, 104, 171

ACOs. *see* Accountable Care Organizations
(ACOs)

acronyms, in training program format, 191

*Advanced Performance Improvement in Health
care* (Lighter), 171

affinity diagram
creating C&E diagram in Analyze
Phase, 119
creating in Define Phase, 50–53
defined, 283

Agency for Healthcare Research and
Quality (AHRQ)
CAHPS Consortium, 29–30
defining clinical practice guidelines,
184–186
patient safety initiatives, 12–13
support for CAHPS surveys, 31

agenda, Kaizen event, 154, 156–157

agile management, 283–284

alpha risk, 126, 284

alternate hypothesis
alpha risk and, 284
beta risk and, 285
defined, 284

**317**

power of an experiment and, 303
reject region and, 307
alternative storage analysis, 6Ss, 161
ambulatory settings, CAPHS survey, 30
American Academy of Family Medicine, 246–247
American Academy of Pediatrics (AAP), 246–247
analysis of variance (ANOVA)
in Analyze Phase, 133–134
assessment of tables, 136–138
example of, 135–136
gauge R&R using, 171
Pocono Medical Center case study using, 219
variants of, 134
analyze, case studies
Miami Baptist Hospital, 216
Nebraska Medical Center, 222
North Shore-Long Island Jewish Health System, 237
Pocono Medical Center, 219
Providence St. Joseph Medical Center, 231, 233
Radia, Inc., 226
Analyze Phase
analysis of variance, 133–138
benefits of, 112–113
brainstorming, 141
cause and effect diagram, 117–120
confidence interval, 131–133
deliverables of, 141–143
discussion questions, 143–144
elements of, 112
essence of, 111–112
hypothesis testing, 125–131
Pearson correlation coefficient, 121–125
references, 144
regression analysis, 138–141
Root Cause Analysis, 113–117
statistical methods of establishing relationships, 120–121
ANOVA. *see* analysis of variance (ANOVA)
appeal process, and Voice of the Customer, 33

approvals, training program, 191
"as-is" process maps, 284
assignable (special) cause
accessing in control charts, 88, 93–94
defined, 284
detecting on run chart, 85–86
overview of, 85
assignable variation, 284
association, causation vs., 122
at risk populations, quality measures for ACOs
COPD, 281
coronary artery disease, 278–279
diabetes, 274–277
frail elderly, 281
heart failure, 277–278
hypertension, 279–280
Attractive quality, Kano Model, 35–39
attributes
defined, 284
ISO framework for quality management, 147
Kano Model, 35–39
attributes data
control chart selection process, 90–93
defined, 284
using IX-MR chart for, 94–95
audit plan, Control Phase, 199–201
autonomation (Jidoka), 153, 285

**B**

background
to performance improvement, 5–8
of project leading to training program, 192
and purpose, Define Phase project charters, 23, 27
and purpose, Improve Phase mini-charters, 150
summarizing problem in brainstorming, 46
background variables, 285
baka yoke, 285
balancing measures, Measure Phase, 101

Baldrige Performance Excellence Program, 200
bar charts
    creating Pareto chart on template for, 83
    Radia, Inc. case study, 226, 228
baseline measures
    calculating analysis of variance, 135–136
    calculating process sigma, 105–107
    defined, 285
    as Measure Phase deliverables, 100
    as Measure Phase goal, 60–61
    Nebraska Medical Center case study,
        221, 223
    NSLIJ case study, 235, 238
    prioritizing in Analyze Phase, 112
    PSMJC case study, 231
    Radia, Inc. case study, 227
benchmarks
    6S event, 160
    ACO financial models, 252–257
    audit plan, 200
    monitoring plan, 195
    National CAHPS benchmarking
        database, 29–31
    pilot test, 167
    quality reporting and improvement, 258
    standardized categories for, 83
best practice, 285
beta risk, 126, 285
Black Belts
    ANOVA testing by, 134
    defined, 285
    NSLIJ Health System case study, 235–236
    project training and mentoring for, 14
    value in Analyze Phase, 112, 121
BNVA (business nonvalue added), 236, 239
brainstorming
    affinity diagrams, 50–53
    in Analyze Phase, 141
    brainwriting and NGT as, 47–48
    C&E diagram, 119–120
    multivoting after, 48–50
    overview of, 46
    prioritization matrix, 74
    procedure for, 46–47

Radia, Inc. case study, 227
    in root cause analysis, 115–116
brainwriting, 47–48
bundled payments, 246, 261
burning platform message, Improve Phase, 148
business nonvalue added (BNVA),
    236, 239

## C
CAHPS Consortium, 29–31
CAHPS Hospital Survey, 30
CAHPS surveys. *see* Consumer Assessment
    of Health Performance Survey
    (CAHPS) surveys
calibration, 286
care coordination, ACOs
    information systems, 269–270
    overview of, 267–269
    transitions, 266–267
case studies. *see* LSS case studies in health care
categories
    5 Whys Analysis, 115
    affinity diagram, 50, 52
    ANOVA test, 134
    healthcare risk adjustment models,
        206–207
    intervals as numeric, 297
    Ishikawa C&E diagram, 117–120, 237
    Kano Model quality, 35–37
    of Measure Phase deliverables, 100–101
    ordered (ordinal), 302
    Pareto chart, 81–83
    run chart, 85
    tracking customer complaint, 32
    unordered (nominal), 302
causation, association vs., 122
cause and effect (C&E) diagram
    Analyze Phase, 117–120
    defined, 286
    NSLIJ Health System case study, 237
c-chart control chart, 88–89
CDHC (consumer driven health care), 6
cellular manufacturing, 286

center line (CL), control charts, 89, 93–94, 286
Centers for Disease Control and Prevention, 29
Centers for Medicare and Medicaid
        Services (CMS)
    Accountable Care Organizations, 251–252
    CAHPS surveys used by, 30
    change in reimbursement policies of, 6–8
    financial models, 252–257
    hospital quality information on Web, 17
    new financial and quality realities, 250
    as part of CAHPS Consortium, 29
    Physicians' Quality Reporting
        Initiative, 245
central tendency, 286
chaku-chaku, 286
champion, 286
change management
    Improve Phase, 148–150
    institutionalization of change, 188–190
charters
    defined, 287
    project, 22–26
checklists
    Control Phase processes, 188–190
    Define Phase processes, 55–56
    PERT statistics, 69
checksheets, 287
CHINs (Community Health Information
        Networks), 248
chi-square tests, case study, 231
CI (confidence interval), 131–133, 287
CL (center line), control charts, 89,
        93–94, 286
clinical practice guidelines (CPGs), 184–187
closure, audit, 201
color codes, 6S, 161
comments, case studies
    Miami Baptist Hospital, 217–218
    Nebraska Medical Center, 223–224
    North Shore-Long Island Jewish Health
        System, 239–240
    Pocono Medical Center, 220
    PSJMC, 233–234
    Radia, Inc., 228

common cause (random) variation
    defined, 287, 306
    indicating in control charts, 88–90,
        202, 226
    indicating on run charts, 83–85
    minimum savings rate in ACOs adjusting
        for, 255–256
    process redesign addressing, 286
    test of significance for, 312
Community Health Information Networks
        (CHINs), 248
*Compendium of Strategies to Prevent
        Healthcare-Associated Infections
        in Acute Care Hospitals* (SHEA
        Web site), 11
complaints, customer, 32–33
computerized provider order entry (CPOE),
        188–189
concurrent review, in managed care, 5–6
confidence interval (CI), 131–133, 287
confidence level, 132–133, 287
confidence limits, 287
confounding, 287
constraints, training program, 193
Consumer Assessment of Health
        Performance Survey (CAHPS)
        surveys
    CAHPS Consortium, 29–30
    CMS, 7–8
    Voice of the Customer, 30–31
consumer driven health care (CDHC), 6
consumers' risk, 287. *see also* beta risk
continuous data
    attributes data vs., 90
    defined, 287
    selecting control charts for, 90–92, 95
continuous quality improvement (CQI),
        Control Phase, 176–177
continuous random variable, 288
continuous-flow production, 287–288
control
    defined, 288
    Miami Baptist Hospital case study, 217
    Nebraska Medical Center case study, 223

North Shore-Long Island Jewish Health
   System case study, 238–239
Pocono Medical Center (PMC) case
   study, 220
PSJMC case study, 232
Radia, Inc. case study, 228
control charts
   in case study, 219
   defined, 288
control charts, Control Phase
   clinical applications, 202–205
   monitoring plan, 195
   risk adjustment, 205
   value of, 201–202
control charts, Measure Phase
   example, 92–93
   interpretation, 93–94
   overview of, 88–90
   selection diagram, 90–92
   tips and tricks, 94–95
Control Phase
   benefits of Analyze Phase to, 113
   control charts, 201–209
   deliverables, 210
   discussion questions, 210–211
   elements of, 176
   essence of, 175–176
   flowcharts, 181–183
   framework for, 176–180
   monitoring plans, 195–201
   NSLIJ Health System case study, 238–239
   other resources, 211–212
   process sigma level, 209–210
   references, 212–213
   risk adjustment, 211–213
   standardization and institutionalization of
      process changes, 183–190
   training plans and programs, 191–195
control specifications, 288
controlled variable, 288
COPD, quality measures for ACOs, 281
coronary artery disease, quality measures for
   ACOs, 278–279
corrective action plan, audit findings, 201

correlation
   in assignable special cause, 284
   defined, 288–289
   not existing in random cause, 306
correlation coefficient, Pearson, 121–125
cost of poor quality (COPQ)
   defined, 289
   increased variation causing, 88
   total, 294
cost reduction
   Miami Baptist Hospital case study, 217
   Nebraska Medical Center case
      study, 223
   North Shore-Long Island Jewish Health
      System case study, 238
   Pocono Medical Center (PMC) case
      study, 220
   PSJMC case study, 232, 234
   Radia, Inc. case study, 227
   in System of Profound Knowledge, 178
   TPS and Six Sigma for, 14–15
CPGs (clinical practice guidelines),
      184–187
Cpk, 289
CPOE (computerized provider order entry),
      188–189
criteria matrix, 289
criterion, prioritization matrix, 74–75
critical path, PERT charts, 64–68
critical X factors
   Analyze Phase focusing on, 143
   case studies, 222, 228
   defined, 61
   design of experiments, 169–170
   project plan, 151
   regression analysis, 138
Critical Y. *see* critical-to-quality (CTQ)
      attributes
Criticality Scores, FMECA, 95–96
critical-to-quality (CTQ) attributes
   in Control Phase, 181–183
   creating tree for, 54–55
   defined, 289
   monitoring plan, 195

overview of, 53–54
PERT charts, 63
in process sigma, 105–107
Critical-to-the-Customer (CTC), 61, 181–183
cross-functional teams, 97, 289
CTC (Critical-to-the-Customer), 61, 181–183
CTQ. *see* critical-to-quality (CTQ) attributes
customer
    defined, 289
    satisfaction surveys, 34–35
customer requirements
    CTC (Critical-to-the-Customer), 61,
        181–183
    defined, 290
    identifying CTQ attributes. *see* critical-to-
        quality (CTQ) attributes
    Kano Model analysis capturing, 39
    quality function deployment related to, 306
    in "should be" process map or
        flowchart, 309
    VOC process capturing. *see* Voice of the
        Customer (VOC)
CUSUM chart, 94
cycle time
    continuous-flow production reducing,
        287–288
    defined, 290
    line balancing equalizing, 299
    manufacturing, 300
    measuring efficiency, 274
    PERT charts determining, 62
    process maps determining, 61
    quick changeover methods for faster, 306
    standard work and, 311

**D**

D (Duration) of step, PERT chart, 63–64
dashboard, 195, 290
data, defined, 290
data collection plan
    defined, 290
    Measure Phase, 100–103
    Voice of the Customer, 29–30
deductible health insurance policies, CDHC, 6

defects, 290
defects per million opportunities (DPMO)
    calculating process sigma, 105–107
    developing High Reliability
        Organization, 177
    measurement system analysis, 105
    overview of, 290–291
define, case studies
    Miami Baptist Hospital, 216
    Nebraska Medical Center, 221
    North Shore-Long Island Jewish Health
        System, 235
    Pocono Medical Center, 218
    PSJMC, 229–230
    Radia, Inc., 225
Define Phase
    affinity diagrams, 50–53
    background, 21–22
    brainstorming, 46–47
    brainwriting and nominal group
        technique, 47–48
    checklist for completion of, 55–56
    critical-to-quality analysis, 53–55
    discussion questions, 56–57
    Kano Model, 35–39
    multivoting, 48–50
    process mapping, 41–44
    project charter, 22–26
    PSJMC case study, 233
    references, 57
    SIPOC process map, 44–45
    stakeholder analysis, 39–41
    Voice of the Customer, 26–30
    Voice of the Customer, listening to, 30–35
degrees of freedom (df)
    calculating ANOVA, 137
    calculating confidence interval, 132
    defined, 291
    t-test, 127, 130
deliverables
    Analyze Phase, 141–143
    Control Phase, 210
    defined, 60
    Improve Phase, 173
    Measure Phase, 100–105

Deming, Edwards
  14 principles for quality improvement,
    178–180
  attractive quality in Kano Model, 35
  value of statistical process control, 88
density function
  defined, 291
  normal distribution as, 302
  parameter of, 303
  t-distribution graph of, 127
departments, breaking down barriers
    between, 179
dependent variables
  assignable (special) cause and, 284
  Control Phase, 183
  defined, 291
  random cause and, 306
  in regression analysis, 138–140
  statistical methods of establishing
    relationships, 120
deployment flowcharts
  defined, 291
  Improve Phase, 163–167
  Measure Phase, 69–72
descriptive statistics, 291
Design for Six Sigma (DFSS), 292
Design of Experiments (DOE), 169–171,
    226, 228
deviation. *see also* standard deviation
  audit plans for trends connoting,
    199–200
  defined, 292
  standard, 310
DFSS (Design for Six Sigma), 292
discrete random variable, 292
discussion questions
  Analyze Phase tools, 143–144
  Control Phase tools, 210–211
  Define Phase tools, 56–57
  LSS case studies in health care, 240–241
  Measure Phase tools, 108–109
  performance improvement, 18–19
distributions, 292
diversity, disparities of healthcare based on,
    247–248

DMADV (Design, Measure, Analyze,
    Design, Verify), 292
DMAIC (Define, Measure, Analyze,
    Improve, and Control)
  Analyze Phase. *see* Analyze Phase
  case studies. *see* LSS case studies in
    health care
  Control Phase. *see* Control Phase
  Define Phase. *see* Define Phase
  defined, 292
  Improve Phase. *see* Improve Phase
  Measure Phase. *see* Measure Phase
  overview of, 16–17
DMAIC (Define, Measure, Analyze, Improve,
    and Control), in reform era
  discussion questions, 262–263
  DMAIC's role as quality improvement
    strategy, 261–262
  financial and quality realities, 250–252
  financial models, 252–257
  health information technology, 260–261
  quality reporting and improvement,
    257–259
  references, 263
  trends in healthcare reform, 243–250
"do no use" list, 11
document history, training program, 191
DOE (Design of Experiments), 169–171,
    226, 228
DPMO. *see* defects per million opportunities
    (DPMO)
Duration (D) of step, PERT chart, 63–64

## E

Earliest Finish (EF) cell, PERT chart, 63–64
Earliest Start (ES) cell, PERT chart, 63
education
  of personnel, 180
  for prevention of mistakes, 196
effectiveness, 292
effects analysis. *see* failure mode and effects
    analysis (FMEA); failure mode
    and effects criticality analysis
    (FMECA)

efficiency
  calculating process cycle efficiency, 76–79
  defined, 292
  gauging process, 24, 44–45
  improving quality of care, 8–10
  ISO system approach to management, 147
  reducing cost with, 14–15
80-20 rule, 81
electronic health records (EHRs), 249, 260
electronic medical records (EMRs), 244, 248
employers, as healthcare payers, 10
ergonomic hazard analysis, 6S, 161
ES (Earliest Start) cell, PERT chart, 63
ethnic disparities, primary care physician
      access, 3–4
evaluation, training program, 192–195
Exact test, 226
Excel
  ANOVA, 134
  bar chart template, 83, 85
  confidence interval, 133
  NSLIJ Health System case study, 238
  Pearson correlation coefficient, 124
executive summary, training program, 191
experimental error, 293
experiments
  analysis of variance, 133–134
  with bundled payments, 246
  defined, 293
  design of experiments (DOE), 169–171
  null hypothesis, 126
  regression analysis, 138, 140
external failure
  cost of poor quality measuring
      impact of, 289
  defined, 293

**F**

F value, ANOVA, 137–138
facilities, training program, 193
factors
  defined, 293
  force field analysis of, 294
  human, 296

failure mode and effects analysis (FMEA)
  case study, 226, 228
  defined, 294
  Improve Phase, 151–152
  monitoring plan in Control Phase, 195
  poka yoke in Control Phase, 196
failure mode and effects criticality analysis
      (FMECA)
  applications of, 95–96
  Measure Phase and, 95
  procedure for, 96–100
failure modes, defined, 95
false positive assessments, control charts, 93–94
F-crit value, ANOVA, 137
fear, employee motivation and, 179
feedback loops, poka yoke, 198
financial and quality realities, 250–252
first-pass yield, 293
Fishbone diagram. *see* cause and effect
      (C&E) diagram
Five (5) Ss, 158, 293–294
Five Whys, 293. *see also* Root Cause
      Analysis (RCA)
fixed effects
  ANOVA variants, 134
  model, 294
flexibility, standardizing health care
      processes, 183–184
flexible manufacturing systems (FMS), 294
flow, defined, 294
flowcharts
  applying to PERT charts, 64
  applying to process cycle efficiency, 76–79
  applying to SIPOC process map, 44–45
  case study using, 232
  conducting Kaizen event, 154
  in Control Phase, 181–183
  creating in Define Phase, 41–44
  deployment, 69–72
FMEA. *see* failure mode and effects analysis
      (FMEA); failure mode and effects
      criticality analysis (FMECA)
FMECA. *see* failure mode and effects
      criticality analysis (FMECA)
FMS (flexible manufacturing systems), 294

focus, Kaizen event, 153
focus groups, Voice of the Customer, 34
force field analysis, 294
forcing functions, poka yoke, 198
Ford, quality emphasis of, 17
formal customer listening methods, 32–33
14 principles for quality improvement,
        178–180
frail elderly, quality measures for
        ACOs, 281
framework
    affinity diagram, 50–53
    audit plan regulatory, 200
    Control Phase, 176–180
    DMADV, 292
    DMAIC. see DMAIC (Define, Measure,
        Analyze, Improve, and Control)
    Improve Phase, 146–147
    measurement system analysis, 103
    project charter, 24–25
    quality, 15–17
frequency distribution, 294, 295


**G**
Gantt chart, 295
gauge, defined, 294
gauge R&R (gauge repeatability and
        reproducibility)
    defined, 294
    Improve Phase, 171
    Measure Phase, 103–105
GDP (gross domestic product), 1–2
General Motors, 10
glossary, training program, 193
goal statement
    defined, 295
    including in charter, 287
    project mini-charter format, 150
government entities, healthcare
        incentives of, 10
Green Belts, 14, 295
grievance process, Voice of the Customer, 33
gross domestic product (GDP), 1–2
Grout, John, 196

**H**
HAIS (hospital acquired infection),
        prevention guidelines, 11
handoffs
    "as-is" process maps with multiple, 284
    cost of poor quality for, 289
    defined, 295
    deployment flowcharts defining, 71–72
    "should be" process maps limiting, 309
Harry, Mikel, 16
Hawthorne effect, 295
H-CAHPS (Hospital CAHPS), 30
Health Effectiveness Data Information Set
        (HEDIS), 7–8, 30
Health Information Exchanges
        (HIEs), 248
Health Information Technology for
        Economic and Clinical Health
        (HITECH) Act, 244
health information technology (HIT),
        260–261
health maintenance organizations (HMOs),
        ranking, 17
Health Outcomes Survey (HOS), 7–8, 30
Health Plan Survey, CAHPS, 30
healthcare accountability circle, 8–9
healthcare costs
    adults with medical bill problems or
        debt, 1, 3
    copayments not covered by Medicare, 3
    managed care and, 5–6
    in US vs. other developed countries, 1–2
HealthGrades Web site, 18
heart failure, quality measures for ACOs,
        277–278
HEDIS (Health Effectiveness Data
        Information Set), 7–8, 30
heijunka, 295
hierarchy of needs, Maslow, 179
HIEs (Health Information Exchanges), 248
High Reliability Organization
        (HRO), 177
histograms, 295
HIT (health information technology),
        260–261

HITECH (Health Information Technology
for Economic and Clinical Health)
Act, 244
home health agencies, comparison of, 17
homeostasis, 148
homogeneity of variance, 295
HOS (Health Outcomes Survey), 7–8, 30
hoshin kanri (policy deployment), 296
hospital acquired infection (HAIs),
prevention guidelines, 11
Hospital CAHPS (H-CAHPS), 30
hospital quality information
CAHPS surveys for, 30–31
on Web, 17–18
HRO (High Reliability Organization), 177
human factors
defined, 296
in gauge R&R, 104
hypertension, quality measures for ACOs,
279–280
hypothesis statement, 296
hypothesis testing
case study, 219
overview of, 125–127
t-test, 128–131

**I**

ICD-10 coding, 244
ICD-9-CM coding, 245
IHI (Institute for Healthcare
Improvement), 13
impact/effort matrix, 296
implementation phase, 6S event, 160–161
implementation plan, 296
improve
Miami Baptist Hospital case study,
216–217
Nebraska Medical Center case study, 222
North Shore-Long Island Jewish Health
System case study, 237–238
Pocono Medical Center (PMC) case
study, 219
PSJMC case study, 231–232
Radia, Inc. case study, 226–227

Improve Phase
6S, 158–162
additional Six Sigma resources, 168–172
benefits of Analyze Phase to, 113
change management, 148–150
completing, 173
Control Phase vs., 176–177
deployment flowcharts, 163–167
discussion questions, 173–174
elements of, 146
essence of, 145–146
failure mode and effects analysis, 151–152
framework for, 146–147
Kaizen, 152–157
pilot testing, 165–168
prioritization matrix, 163
project plan, 150–151
Radia, Inc. case study, 227
references, 174
training program, 191
improvement, defined, 296
incentives, performance-based provider,
245–246
independent variables
defined, 296
design of experiments, 169
factors as, 293
Pearson correlation coefficient, 125
primary control variables in experiment
as, 304
regression analysis, 138–139
Indifferent quality, Kano Model, 36–39
Individual X-Moving Range (IX-MR) chart,
94–95, 239
infant mortality rate, 1–2
infection control, 11, 200
informal customer listening methods, 32–34
information, multiple sources of health, 247
Institute for Healthcare Improvement
(IHI), 13
Institute of Medicine (IOM), 246–247
institutionalization of process change,
Control Phase, 188–190
insurers, healthcare incentives of, 10
interaction, 297

internal rate of return (IRR), 297
International Organization for
        Standardization (ISO), Improve
        Phase, 146–147
Internet sites on health care
    health information technology, 260
    improved quality of care for patients, 8–9
    recent trend in, 247
intervals
    analyzing continuous data at, 90
    confidence interval, 131–133, 255
    defined, 297
    systematic sampling at fixed time, 312
    variables data measured at, 314
inventory
    6S in lab setting, 159
    continuous-flow production slashing,
        287–288
    poka yoke in Control Phase, 199
    setting aside specific, 308
    waste associated with, 301
    work-in-process inventory, 315
IOM (Institute of Medicine), 246–247
Ishikawa diagram. *see* cause and effect
        (C&E) diagram

**J**
Jidoka (autonomation), 153, 285, 303–304
Job 1, quality as, 17–18
just-in-time (JIT), 152, 297

**K**
kaikaku, 297
Kaizen
    conducting Kaizen event, 153–157
    defined, 297
    in Improve Phase, 152
    management principles, 152–153
Kaizen event
    case study, 235–240
    conducting, 153–157
    defined, 152, 297
    management principles, 152–153

kanban
    overview of, 298
    pull system using, 305
    using visual cues and signage to reduce
        errors, 198–199
kanban signals, 298
kano analysis, 298
Kano Model, 35–39
karoshi, 298
key performance indicators (KPIs), 173, 299
Kirkpatrick Learning and Training
        Evaluation model, 194–195

**L**
Latest Finish cell, PERT chart, 63
Latest Start cell, PERT chart, 63–64
lead time
    defined, 299
    process cycle efficiency calculation, 76
    processing time as small fraction of, 305
leadership
    conducting Kaizen events, 155
    motivating teams, 178
    shaping performance, 179
    supporting Control Phase, 188
lean manufacturing or lean production, 299
level scheduling, 299, 301
life cycle costing, 299
Likert scale
    prioritization matrix, 74, 76
    stakeholder analysis, 41
    utilizing t-test for comparing samples, 131
line balancing, 299, 301
line charts, 83, 299
linear regression, 138–141
linear relationships, Pearson correlation
        coefficient, 124–125
lower control limit
    control charts, 88–89, 94
    defined, 299
    X-bar and R chart, 315
LSS case studies in health care
    discussion questions, 240–241
    Miami Baptist Hospital, 216–218

Nebraska Medical Center, 221–224
North Shore-Long Island Jewish Health
    System, 234–240
overview of, 215–216
Pocono Medical Center, 218–220
Providence St. Joseph Medical Center,
    229–234
Radia, Inc., 224–228
references, 241

# M

machine availability rate, 299–300
managed care, 5–6, 207
management by objective, eliminating, 179
manufacturing cells, 300
manufacturing cycle time, 300
Maslow, Abraham, 179
Master Black Belts, 14, 300
materials, training program, 193
maximum sharing percentage (MSP),
    financial models, 256
Mean Square (MS), ANOVA tables,
    137–138
Meaningful Use criteria, EMRs, 244, 260
measure
    defined, 300
    Miami Baptist Hospital case study, 216
    Nebraska Medical Center case study, 221
    North Shore-Long Island Jewish Health
        System case study, 236
    NSLIJ Health System case study, 236
    Pocono Medical Center (PMC) case
        study, 218
    PSJMC case study, 230–231
    Radia, Inc. case study, 225–226
Measure Phase
    calculating process sigma, 105–107
    deliverables in, 100–105
    deployment flowchart, 69–72
    discussion questions, 108–109
    essence of, 59–61
    finishing, 107
    overview of, 60

PERT charts. *see* Program Evaluation and
    Review Technique (PERT) charts
prioritization matrix, 72–76
process cycle efficiency, 76–79
process maps, 61–62
references, 108
time value analysis. *see* time value analysis
    (TVA)
measurement system analysis, gauge R&R,
    103–105, 171
measuring instruments, gauge R&R, 104
medical errors
    goal of patient safety, 10–14
    mistake proofing with poka yoke,
        196–199
    Pareto chart application to, 82–83
    Swiss cheese model of error propagation,
        113–114
Medicare Shared Savings program
    benchmark and target savings in ACOs,
        252–253
    new financial realities, 251–252
    PQRS bonus eligibility, 259
    tracks for shared savings in ACOs,
        253–255
medication ordering, 11
metrics, pilot testing in Improve Phase,
    167–168
Miami Baptist Hospital case study, 216–218
Microsoft Project, for PERT charts, 64, 68
Microsoft Visio®
    for cause and effect diagram, 119
    for deployment flowchart, 69–72
    for PERT chart, 64–67
    for process flowchart, 42
    for SIPOC process map, 44–45
mini-charter, project plan, 150–151
minimum savings rate (MSR), financial
    models, 255–256
mission statement
    policies consistent with, 184–185
    project charter, 23, 25
mistake proofing (poka yoke), 196–199, 303
mixed-model production, 300

monitoring plan
  audit plan, 199–201
  case study, 228
  elements of, 195–196
  poka yoke, 196–199
Morbidity and Mortality Rounds on the
    Web, AHRQ, 13
motion, muda (waste), 301
MS (Mean Square), ANOVA tables, 137–138
MSP (maximum sharing percentage),
    financial models, 256
MSR (minimum savings rate), financial
    models, 255–256
muda (waste)
  case study, 236, 239
  defined, 300
  kaikaku eliminating, 297
  kaizen creating more value with less, 297
  overproduction as, 300
  reducing cost, 14–15
  standard work as most free of, 311
multiple regression
  ANOVA as, 134
  based on linear regression, 138
  case study, 219
  defined, 301
  in regression analysis, 140–142
multivoting, 48–50, 301
mura, 301. *see also* variation
muri, 301
Must-be quality, Kano Model, 36–39

# N

nagara, 301
National CAHPS Benchmarking Database,
    29, 31
National Committee for Quality Assurance
    (NCQA), 30
National Institute for Disability and
    Rehabilitation Research, 29
National Patient Safety Goals (NPSGs),
    11–12
natural mapping, poka yoke, 198

NCQA (National Committee for Quality
    Assurance), 30
Nebraska Medical Center Peggy D. Cowdery
    Patient Care Center case study,
    221–224
negative scores, prioritization matrix, 74
nemawashi, 301
newsletter, CAHPS Connection, 31
NGT (nominal group technique), 47–48
"no blame" safety reporting Web sites, 12
nominal, 302
nominal group technique (NGT), 47–48
nonconforming unit, 302
nonconformity, 302
nonlinear relationships, 124–125
nonvalue added (NVA) work
  case study, 228, 236–237, 239
  defined, 302
  TVA chart, 79–80
normal distribution
  confidence interval, 132
  control charts, 88
  defined, 302
  t-test, 127
North Carolina Hospital Quality
    Performance Report Web site, 18
North Shore-Long Island Jewish (NSLIJ)
    Health System case study
  analyze, 237
  comments, 239–240
  control, 238–239
  cost reduction, 238
  define, 235
  improve, 237–238
  measure, 236
  problem statement, 234
  quality metric changes, 238
  references, 240
Notice of Proposed Rule Making (NPRM)
  Accountable Care Organizations, 250–252
  financial models, 252–257
  Meaningful Use, 260
  quality reporting and improvement,
    257–259

NPRM. *see* Notice of Proposed Rule Making (NPRM)

NPSGs (National Patient Safety Goals), 11–12

NSLIJ. *see* North Shore-Long Island Jewish (NSLIJ) Health System case study

null hypothesis
defined, 302
hypothesis testing, 126–131
procedure for t-test, 128–130

nursing homes, CMS comparison of, 17

NVA. *see* nonvalue added (NVA) work


## O

Office of the National Coordinator of Health Information Technology (ONCHIT), 248

ONCHIT (Office of the National Coordinator of Health Information Technology), 248

One-dimensional quality, Kano Model, 36–39

one-sided alternative, 302

one-sided models, ACOs, 253–256, 259

one-tailed t-test, 127–130

online journals, AHRQ, 12

online resources
Agency for Healthcare Research and Quality (AHRQ), 12–13
CAHPS survey results, 30
CAHPS User Network, 31
Clinical Practice Guideline Clearinghouse, 186
comparing healthcare entities, 17–18
Institute for Healthcare Improvement, 13
Society for Epidemiology of America, 11

operational definitions, 101–103, 302

operational framework, project charter, 24–25

ordinal, 302

output/outcome measures
defined, 302
monitoring plan, 195

pilot test, 167
process metrics in Measure Phase, 100–101

overproduction, muda (waste), 300

ownership, patient clinical record information, 248–249


## P

P chart
case study, 228
control chart selection, 91
defined, 303

P&Ps (policies and procedures), 184–185

parameters
defined, 303
one-sided alternative value of, 302

Pareto charts
applied to medical errors, 82–83
case study, 219, 226, 228
defined, 303
overview of, 80–81
tips and tricks, 83

Pareto principle, 80–81

Part D drug plans (PDPs), 17

participants, brainstorming, 47

patient clinical record information, ownership of, 248–250

Patient Protection and Affordable Care Act (PPACA) of 2010
Accountable Care Organization, 250–252
DMAIC and, 261–262
trends in healthcare reform. *see* trends in healthcare reform

patient safety
goal of, 10–14
quality measures for ACOs, 270

patient/caregiver experience, quality measures for ACOs, 266

patient-centered medical home (PCMH), 246–247

patients
goal of patient safety, 10–14
healthcare incentives of, 8–9

payers, healthcare incentives of, 10

PCE (process cycle efficiency), 76–79
PCMH (patient-centered medical home),
    246–247
PDCA (Plan-Do-Check-Act), 145
PDCA (Plan-Do-Check-Act) cycle, 15–17
PDPs (Part D drug plans), 17
PDSA (Plan-Do-Study-Act) cycle, 303
Pearson correlation coefficient, 121–125
performance
    monitoring plan targets, 195
    project charter content, 24–25
performance, audit, 200
performance improvement
    background, 5–8
    cost reduction, 14–15
    discussion questions, 18–19
    patient safety, 10–14
    quality as Job 1, 17–18
    quality frameworks, 15–17
    quality of care, 8–10
    references, 19–20
    US Health System Performance
        scorecard, 1–5
performance-based incentives for providers,
    245–246
personal health records (PHRs), 249–250
PHRs (personal health records), 249–250
physician quality reporting system
    (PQRS), 259
physicians
    healthcare incentives of, 9–10
    variation in access to primary care, 3–4
Physicians' Quality Reporting Initiative
    (PQRI), 245
pilot testing, 165–168
Plan-Do-Check-Act (PDCA), 145
Plan-Do-Check-Act (PDCA) cycle, 15–17
planning phase
    6S events, 159–160
    audits, 200
PLT (Production Lead Time), PCE
    calculation, 76
PMC (Pocono Medical Center) case study,
    218–220

Pocono Medical Center (PMC) case study,
    218–220
poka yoke (mistake proofing), 196–199, 303
policies and procedures (P&Ps), 184–185
policy deployment (hoshin kanri), 296
population. see also at risk populations,
        quality measures for ACOs
    ACO financial models for, 252–256
    calculating confidence interval
        for, 131–133
    clinical applications of control
        charts, 202–205
    defined, 303
    descriptive statistics defining, 291
    histogram displaying distribution of, 295
    hypothesis testing on, 125–131
    pilot testing on smaller subset of, 165–168
    random sampling of, 306
    sample of, 289
    selecting risk adjustment model for, 208
    subgroup of, 311
    systematic sampling of, 312
population standard deviation ($\sigma$),
        confidence interval, 132–133
post-implementation phase, 6S events,
    160–161
power of an experiment, 303
PPACA. see Patient Protection and Affordable
        Care Act (PPACA) of 2010
PQRI (Physicians' Quality Reporting
        Initiative), 245
PQRS (physician quality reporting
        system), 259
precision, 104, 303
preventive health, quality measures for
        ACOs, 270–274
preventive screenings, and high deductible
        plans, 6
pride of workmanship, 180
primary care physicians
    ethic disparity in accessing, 3–4
    patient-centered medical homes and,
        246–247
    satisfaction with medical practice, 3–4

primary control variables, 304

prior authorization, managed care, 5–6

prioritization

    conducting Kaizen event, 153–154

    using brainstorming. *see* brainstorming

prioritization matrix (PM)

    conducting Kaizen event, 154

    in Improve Phase, 163–164

    in Measure Phase, 72–76

probability

    alpha risk, 285

    beta risk, 285

    clinical data tracking using control
        chart, 205

    confidence level, 287

    consumers' risk, 287

    defined, 304

    density function, 291

    power of an experiment, 303

    producers' risk, 305

    run chart table of, 86

    t-test distribution, 127–130

probability of an event, 304

problem, defining in brainstorming, 46

problem statement

    Miami Baptist Hospital case study, 216

    Nebraska Medical Center case study, 221

    North Shore-Long Island Jewish Health
        System case study, 234

    Pocono Medical Center (PMC) case
        study, 218

    PSJMC case study, 229

    Radia, Inc. case study, 224

procedures, standardizing, 184–185

process, 304

process average, 304

process capability, 304

process cycle efficiency (PCE), 76–79

process management

    defined, 304

    ISO framework for continual
        improvement, 147

    reducing cost with lean, 14

    throughput as classical problem of lean, 239

process maps

    case study, 231

    creating in Define Phase, 41–44

    defined, 304

    for deployment flowchart, 69–72

    refining in Measure Phase, 61–62

    SIPOC, 44–45

process metrics

    audit plan, 200

    monitoring plan, 195

    with operational definitions, 100–103

    pilot testing, 167

process owners

    audit plan and, 200–201

    as brainstorming participant, 47

    deployment flowchart for, 69–72, 165

    feedback during pilot test from, 165

    feedback on process flowchart from, 43

    monitoring plan and, 195

    monitoring plan identifying, 195

    transfer of project ownership to, 210

process redesign, 85, 304

process shift, 85

process sigma

    calculating, 105–107

    NSLIJ Health System case study, 236

process sigma level, 209–210

process spread, 305

processing, muda (waste), 301

processing time, 305

producers' risk, 305

Production Lead Time (PLT), PCE
    calculation, 76

productivity, constantly improving, 178

products, building quality into, 178

Program Evaluation and Review Technique
    (PERT) charts

    creating in Measure Phase, 62–64

    putting statistics in deployment
        flowcharts, 72

    steps in creating, 64–68

    tips and tricks, 69

    using for PCE calculation, 76–79

project, 305

project charter
  purposes of, 22–23
  structure and content of, 23–26
  template, 27–29
project plan, Improve Phase, 150–151
Providence St. Joseph Medical Center
        (PSJMC) case study
  analyze, 231
  comments, 233–234
  control, 232
  cost reduction, 232
  define, 229–230
  improve, 231–232
  measure, 230–231
  problem statement, 229
  quality metric changes, 232
  references, 234
providers
  Accountable Care Organization, 250–252
  performance-based incentives for, 245–246
P/T ratio, gauge R&R, 104–105
pull, 305
pull system, 287–288, 305
p-value
  ANOVA, 136–137
  level of confidence in hypothesis testing,
        126–127
  multiple regression, 141–142
  t-test procedure, 129, 131

**Q**

QFD (quality function deployment), 305–306
QI framework. *see* quality improvement
        (QI) framework
QI Macros
  creating ANOVA models, 134
  creating control chart, 90
  creating PERT chart, 82–83
quality function deployment (QFD),
        305–306
quality improvement (QI) framework
  14 principles for quality improvement,
        178–180

overview of, 15–17
  role of DMAIC as, 261–262
quality metric changes
  Miami Baptist Hospital case study, 217
  Nebraska Medical Center case study,
        222–223
  North Shore-Long Island Jewish Health
        System case study, 238
  Pocono Medical Center (PMC) case
        study, 219
  PSJMC case study, 232
  Radia, Inc. case study, 227
quality of care
  goal of patient safety, 10–14
  improving, 8–10
  Medicare incentive program, 6–8
quick changeover methods, 306

**R**

R (range control) chart
  control charts, 202–203, 205
  defined, 306, 315
Radia, Inc. case study
  analyze, 226
  comments, 228
  control, 228
  cost reduction, 227
  define, 225
  improve, 226–227
  measure, 225–226
  problem statement, 224
  quality metric changes, 227
  references, 228
random, defined, 306
random cause, 306
random sample
  defined, 306
  difficulty of obtaining, 131–132
  utilizing ANOVA, 135
random variable
  confidence level and, 287
  continuous, 288
  defined, 306

density function of, 291
discrete, 292
random variation, 306
randomized control trial (RCT), 169–171
range, defined, 306
rapid cycle improvement, Kaizen event,
    152–153
rating systems, eliminating personnel,
    179–180
RCT (randomized control trial), 169–171
red tag system, 6S, 161
references
    Analyze Phase, 144
    Control Phase, 211–213
    Define Phase, 57
    LSS case studies in health care, 241
    Measure Phase, 108
    Miami Baptist Hospital case study, 218
    Nebraska Medical Center case study, 224
    North Shore-Long Island Jewish Health
        System case study, 240
    performance improvement, 19–20
    personal health record programs, 249
    Pocono Medical Center (PMC) case
        study, 220
    PSJMC case study, 234
    Radia, Inc. case study, 228
Regional Health Information Organizations
    (RHIOs), 248
regression analysis
    example of, 140–142
    multiple regression, 140–141
    overview of, 138
    simple linear regression, 138–140
reimbursement, ACO model of, 250–252
reject region, 307
relationships
    building high quality business, 178
    statistical methods of establishing. *see*
        statistical methods of establishing
        relationships
repeatability, gauge R&R, 103–105
reporting, audit, 201
representative sample, 307

reproducibility, gauge R&R, 103–105
requirements, training program, 192
resistance to change, Improve Phase, 148
retroactive denials, managed care, 5–6
return on investment (ROI)
    defined, 307
    Pareto chart demonstrating, 81
    stakeholder analysis, 39
Reverse quality, Kano Model, 36–39
reverse Root Cause Analysis, 151–152
review team, prioritization matrix, 74
rework, muda (waste), 301
rework loop, 307
risk adjustment models, Control Phase
    example use of, 207
    overview of, 205–207
    resources for, 212
    selection of, 208–209
Risk Priority Number (RPN), FMECA
    process, 96–98, 100
robust, 307
roles and responsibilities, training program
    staff, 192
rolled throughput yield (RTY), 307
root cause analysis (RCA)
    Analyze Phase, 113–117
    applying poka yoke in Control Phase, 196
    case study, 231
    on control charts, 88, 93–94
    defined, 307
    FMECA as form of reverse,
        95–100, 151–152
    monitoring plan role, 195
    for special cause variation, 85
RPN (Risk Priority Number), FMECA
    process, 96–98, 100
rules, control chart interpretation, 94
run charts
    control charts as version of. *see*
        control charts
    defined, 83, 307
    procedure for, 83–86
    in time value analysis, 83–88
    tips and tricks, 87–88

## S

S (Slack) times, PERT charts, 63, 68, 78
Safety, 6S
  defined, 158
  evaluation form, 162
  improvement tool(s) for, 161
  lab setting example, 159
safety, goal of patient
  initiatives, 11–13
  overview of, 10–11
  Six Sigma approach to, 13–14
safety audits, 200
sample, 307
sample size (n), confidence interval formula, 132–133
sampling bias, 307–308
satisfaction metrics, pilot testing, 167
scatterplots
  defined, 308
  in linear regression, 139–140
  in Pearson correlation coefficient, 121–125
scheduling
  level, 299
  NSLIJ Health System case study, 237–238
SCHIP (State Children's Health Insurance Program), 30
SCIP 3 metric. *see* Providence St. Joseph Medical Center (PSJMC) case study
scope
  defined, 308
  Kaizen event, 153–154
  project charter, 24–25
  training program, 192
scoring, prioritization matrix, 74–76
SDN (self-directed natural work teams), 308
seasonal adjustment, control charts, 202–203
seiban, 308
seiketsu, 5Ss, 294
seiri, 5Ss, 293
seison, 5Ss, 293
seiton, 5Ss, 293
self-actualization, quality improvement, 179–180

self-directed natural work teams (SDN), 308
self-improvement programs, personnel, 180
sensei, 308
service, improving quality of, 178
sessions, training program, 192
setup times
  continuous-flow production reducing, 287
  defined, 308
  quick changeover methods reducing, 306
seven quality tools, 309
SHEA (Society for Epidemiology of America), 11
Shine, 5Ss, 293
Shine, 6Ss
  defined, 158
  evaluation form, 162
  example in lab setting, 159
  improvement tool(s) for, 161
shitsuke, 5Ss, 294
"Should Be" process map or flowchart, 309
sigma levels, control charts, 89–90, 94
sigma value
  calculating DPMO to determine, 106–107
  defined, 309
signal, 298, 309
simple linear regression, 138–140, 309
single piece flow
  cycle time and, 290
  defined, 310
  eliminating muda with, 297
  implementing with chaku-chaku, 286
  manufacturing cells supporting, 300
  nagara as, 301
  requiring few kanban, 298
SIPOC (Suppliers, Inputs, Process, Outputs, and Customers) process map
  case study, 225–226, 228
  creating, 44–45
  defined, 310
  in Improve Phase, 171–172
Six (6) Ss
  applying poka yoke, 198
  conducting 6S event, 159–162
  defined, 293–294

example in lab setting, 159
overview of, 158
workplace principles, 158–162
Six Sigma
Analyze Phase. *see* Analyze Phase
Control Phase. *see* Control Phase
Define Phase. *see* Define Phase
defined, 310
development of, 16
fundamental equation as basis of, 61
healthcare cost reduction using, 14–15
improvement tools, 168–172
Measure Phase. *see* Measure Phase
patient safety, 13–14
process sigma, 105–107
Slack (S) times, PERT charts, 63, 68, 78
Smith, Bill, 16
Society for Epidemiology of America
(SHEA), 11
Sort, 5Ss, 293
Sort, 6Ss
defined, 158
evaluation form, 162
example in lab setting, 159
improvement tool(s) for, 161
sources of variation, ANOVA tables, 136
spaghetti chart, 310
SPC. *see* statistical process control (SPC)
Speak up program, TJC, 11–12
special cause. *see* assignable (special) cause
SS (Sum of Squares), ANOVA, 137
stakeholders
analyzing in Define Phase, 39–41
change management process and,
148–149
creating deployment flowchart
for, 69–72
defined, 310
monitoring plan identifying, 195
standard deviation
defined, 310
included in descriptive statistics, 273
variance as square of, 314
Z scores and, 316

standard operating procedure
overview of, 310–311
as part of implementation plan, 296
standard work, 311
standardization of process changes
clinical practice guidelines, 184–187
concept of, 183–184
defined, 183
policies and procedures, 184–185
quality assurance checklists, 188
Standardize, 5Ss
defined, 158, 293
evaluation form, 162
example in lab setting, 159
improvement tool(s) for, 161
standards, audit plan, 200
Star Ratings report, 6–7, 30
State Children's Health Insurance Program
(SCHIP), 30
statistical control, 311
statistical methods of establishing
relationships
ANOVA, 133–138
confidence interval, 131–133
hypothesis testing, 125–131
overview of, 120–121
Pearson correlation coefficient, 121–125
regression analysis, 138–141
statistical process control (SPC)
creating control charts. *see* control charts
creating run charts, 85
defined, 311
storyboard, 311
Straighten, 5Ss, 293
Straighten, 6Ss
defined, 158
evaluation form, 162
example in lab setting, 159
improvement tool(s) for, 161
strategy, training program, 192
stratification, 311
stratified frequency plots, case study, 219
subgroups, 91, 311
subprocesses, 312

Sum of Squares (SS), ANOVA, 137
support requirements, project charter, 23, 26
surveillance, audit plans as health care,
    199–200
Sustain, 5S, 293
Sustain, 6S
    defined, 158
    evaluation form, 162
    example in lab setting, 159
    improvement tool(s) for, 161
Swiss cheese model of error propagation,
    113–114
symbols, flowchart, 42–43
System of Profound Knowledge, 178–180
systematic sampling, 312

# T
table of contents, training program, 191
takt time, 312
TapRooT system, 114
tax identification numbers (TINs), ACOs, 251
teams
    conducting Kaizen event, 153–157,
        236–240
    Kaizen event principle of empowering, 152
    role in 6S events, 158
    role in change management, 148–149
    role in project charter, 24–25
    role in root cause analysis, 115
TeamSTEPPS™ National Training
    Network, 13
templates
    Excel® bar chart, 83
    FMECA data, 99
    project charter, 27–29
    SIPOC process map, 44–45
    tracking spreadsheet, 154–155
    training program development, 193
test methods, gauge R&R, 104–105
test of significance, 312
The Joint Commission (TJC), 11–12, 18
The Leapfrog Group Web site, 18
Theory of Constraints, 217

throughput time
    defined, 312
    problem of. *see* North Shore-Long Island
        Jewish (NSLIJ) Health System
        case study
    processing time as small fraction of, 305
    relationship of lead time to, 299
time sequence, process flowcharts, 42
time series plots
    case study, 219, 231
    run charts, 84, 87
time value analysis (TVA)
    control charts, 88–95
    FMECA and, 95–100
    overview of, 79–80
    Pareto charts, 80–83
    run charts, 83–88
times
    PCE calculation, 78
    PERT charts and, 63–68
TINs (tax identification numbers),
    ACOs, 251
Tips for consumers and patients, AHRQ, 13
TJC (The Joint Commission), 11–12, 18
*To Err is Human: Building a Safer Health Care
    System* (Institute of Medicine),
    10–11
tolerance levels, gauge R&R, 104–105
tollgates (or gates), 312
total cost of poor quality, 312
Total Productive Maintenance (TPM)
    programs, 312–313
Total Quality Control (TQC), 313
Total Quality Management (TQM), 313
Toyota Production System (TPS),
    14–15, 114–115
TPM (Total Productive Maintenance)
    programs, 312–313
TPS (Toyota Production System),
    14–15, 114–115
tracking, conducting Kaizen event, 154–155
training
    applying poka yoke, 196
    conducting Kaizen event, 154

institute on the job, 178
plans and programs in Control Phase,
191–195
workarounds as result of ineffective, 189
transportation, muda (waste), 300
tree diagrams
cause and effect, 117–120
control chart selection decision, 91–95
critical-to-quality, 54–55, 181–182
defined, 313
trend charts, 85–86, 195
trends, detecting special cause, 85
trends in healthcare reform
disparities based on diversity, 247–248
Health Information Exchanges, 248
ICD-10 coding, 245
Meaningful Use criteria for EMRs, 244
multiple sources of health information, 247
overview of, 243–244
ownership of patient clinical records,
248–249
patient-centered medical home, 246–247
performance-based incentives for
providers, 245–246
Physicians' Quality Reporting Initiative, 245
value-based purchasing, 244
t-test
ANOVA testing vs., 133
case study, 226
example, 131
in hypothesis testing, 126–127
procedure for, 128–130
usefulness in Analyze Phase, 131
two-sided models, ACOs
financial risk, 255–257
quality reporting and improvement, 259
two-tailed t-tests, 127–131
Type I error. *see* alpha risk
Type II error. *see* beta risk

**U**

Universal Protocol, 12
updates, change management process, 148

upper control limit
in control charts, 88–89, 94
defined, 313
in X-bar and R charts, 315
US Health System Performance scorecard,
19–20
User Network, CAHPS, 29, 31

**V**

value, defined, 313
value, policies consistent with organizational,
184–185
value added activities, 313
value added (VA) ratio
case study, 236, 239
PCE calculation, 76–79
TVA chart, 79–80
value stream, 314
value stream mapping (VSM), 76–79, 314
value-based purchasing (VBP)
building high quality relationships, 178
clinical practice guidelines for, 186
trends in healthcare reform, 244
variables
background, 285
confounding, 287
continuous random, 288
controlled, 288
correlation between, 288–289
defined, 314
dependent, 291
discrete random, 292
parameters, 303
primary control, 304
random. *see* random variable
statistical methods of establishing
relationships between, 120–121
using ANOVA to test multiple, 133–138
variables data, 314
variance
analysis of variance. *see* analysis of variance
(ANOVA)
defined, 314

descriptive statistics defining, 291
homogeneity of, 295
indicating on control chart, 311
process spread encompassing, 305
special cause, 88
variation
accessing in control charts. *see* control charts
common cause, 85
defined, 314
mura as, 301
special cause, 85–86
VBP. *see* value-based purchasing (VBP)
visibility, in poka yoke, 198
Visio®. *see* Microsoft Visio®
vision statement, 184–185
visual control, 314
visual work instructions, 6S, 161
visual workplace, 314
Voice of the Business (VOB), 315
Voice of the Customer (VOC)
with CAHPS surveys, 30–31
case study, 235
data collection methods, 29–30
defined, 315
with other methods, 32–35
overview of, 26
voting system, prioritization matrix, 74
VSM (value stream mapping), 76–79, 314

**W**

waiting, muda (waste), 300
waste, 315. *see also* muda (waste)
weight numbers, prioritization
matrix, 74–75
weighted score, prioritization matrix, 74–76
WIP (work-in-process inventory), 315
work relative value units (WRVUs), 189
workarounds
Kaizen event agenda, 156
monitoring plan preventing, 195
process map revealing, 43–44
as result of ineffective training, 189
root cause analysis factors, 116

workforce
14 principles for quality improvement
of, 178–180
in cause and effect diagram, 119
in high functioning organizations, 147
institutionalization of change for,
188–190
Kaizen events empowering, 152
standardizing process change for, 183–190
training plans and programs for, 191–195
work-in-process inventory (WIP), 315
workplace
14 principles for quality improvement, 180
institutionalizing change in, 188
utilizing 6S in, 158–162, 198
utilizing Kaizen in, 152–157
visual, 314
WRVUs (work relative value units), 189

**X**

X factors. *see* critical X factors
X-bar and R chart, 91, 315

**Y**

Y metric
CTQ attributes. *see* critical-to-quality
(CTQ) attributes
Measure Phase, 61
yamazumi, 315
Yellow Belts, 315
yield
defined, 315
first-pass, 293
on investment, 297
rolled throughput yield, 307
yield improvement, 196, 316

**Z**

Z value, confidence interval formula,
132–133
Z-score (standard scores), 316